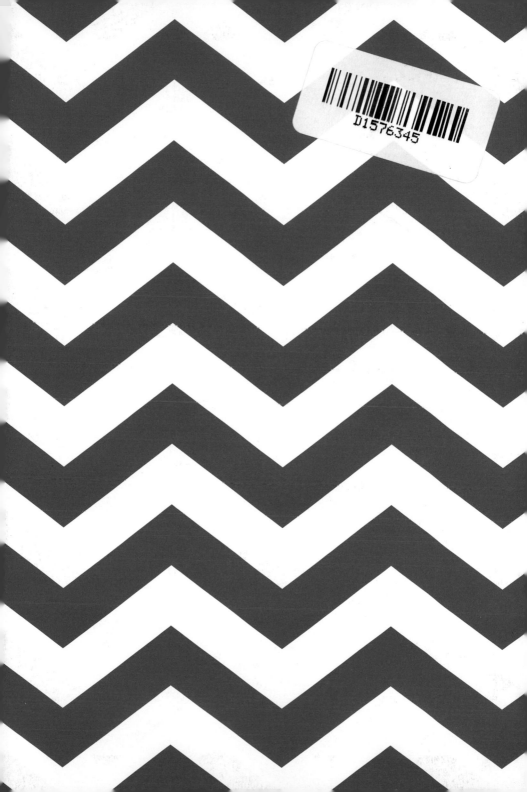

MOTHERHOOD. THE JOURNEY IS YOUR OWN.

The journey of a mother is an epic one. Raising a small person (or people) is such a joy and privilege, but every mum sometimes needs a little encouragement or a moment of reflection.

The Not-So-New Mum's Notebook written by Amy Ransom – mum of three – is the follow-up to the popular first instalment, *The New Mum's Notebook.*

The Not-So-New Mum's Notebook will take you beyond the first year of life with your child up until the moment they're ready to start school, giving you a place to celebrate all of your victories, no matter how small. It will prompt you to think about *yourself* whilst caring for others and help you to remember, in years to come, how you felt and just how brilliant your toddler or preschooler was.

With pages and pages of reassurance, self-care and space to write down all your thoughts and memories, *The Not-So-New Mum's Notebook* will make you feel good about yourself – and about how you're *already* raising your child. Think of it as that friend who always has an empathetic or cheering word when you need it most.

You're a great mum. Just as you are.

ALSO BY AMY RANSOM

The New Mum's Notebook – a reassuring, funny and down-to-earth companion to the first year.

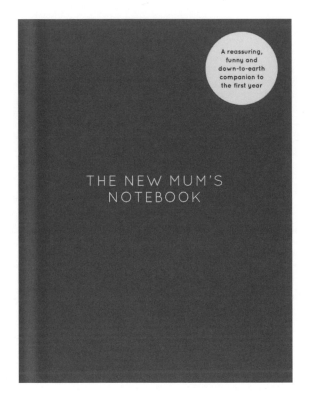

A reassuring, funny and down-to-earth companion to the first year

THE NEW MUM'S NOTEBOOK

GET IN TOUCH

Share and tag your photos of
The Not-So-New Mum's Notebook
#TheNotSoNewMumsNotebook

Get in touch:
www.amyransom.com
Facebook.com/amyransomwrites
Instagram.com/amyransomwrites
Twitter.com/amyransomwrites

THE NOT-SO-NEW MUM'S NOTEBOOK

A journal for the toddler and preschool years

Amy Ransom

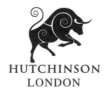

HUTCHINSON
LONDON

1 3 5 7 9 10 8 6 4 2

Hutchinson
20 Vauxhall Bridge Road
London SW1V 2SA

Hutchinson is part of the Penguin Random House group of companies whose
addresses can be found at global.penguinrandomhouse.com.

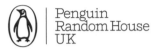

Penguin
Random House
UK

Illustration credits: p.42 © marcin jucha/Shutterstock Images. p.66 © PHB.cz
(Richard Semik)/Shutterstock Images. p.66 © alisafarov/Shutterstock Images. p.168
© Ekaterina Kondratova/Shutterstock Images. p.214 © Infinity Time/Shutterstock
Images. p.215 © ffolas/Shutterstock Images. All other images courtesy of Amy
Ransom. 'Moonflower' typeface © Denise Bentulan

First published in the United Kingdom by Hutchinson in 2018

www.penguin.co.uk

A CIP catalogue record for this book is available from the British Library.

ISBN 9781786331175

Printed and bound in Italy by L.E.G.O. S.P.A.

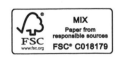

For my tribe, Eva, Ivy and Joseph.
Thank you for trusting me to shape your
wonderful little minds.

And to every amazing not-so-new mum out there.
Always remember: the journey is your own.

Contents

me and you

Who I am..

Who you are..

How old you were when I started this notebook ....

What I thought when I started this notebook ....

....

....

One thing I wish for you ....

....

One thing I wish for myself ....

....

Dear Not-So-New Mum,

Firstly, it's so lovely to see you. Thank you so much for allowing me to be a small part of your motherhood journey.

If you've joined me from the first instalment – *The New Mum's Notebook* – you'll have an idea of what to expect here. If, on the other hand, you've arrived straight here with a toddler, threenager or preschooler in tow, hello and get stuck in! No matter what your child's age, this is your book to use from the beginning, as frequently as you like. Use the contents page to dip in and out, as we all reach stages at different times. I hope you find everything you need to navigate the early years amidst these reassuring articles, affirmations and pages of journal space. Keeping a note of your thoughts, feelings and memories is now widely acknowledged by psychologists as being so beneficial for our well-being. There is nothing quite like looking back on all that you have overcome – and loved – to give you the strength to keep going. Enjoy using the prompts in the top right-hand column of the double journal pages, to contemplate all the stuff that matters to YOU.

The Not-So-New Mum's Notebook is for all you Not-So-New mums during those wonderfully funny, but often tricky, early years from one to four/five, before your child starts school. This is NOT a parenting book: giving advice is such a grey area and I'm not sure anyone is ever *really* qualified to give it, because no one knows you or your child as you do.

I wish I had known this when my first baby was eight weeks old and I found myself standing in the baby-book aisle of my local bookshop, searching desperately for the answer to motherhood. Actually, I was looking for the answer to how to get some sleep (for the baby and me), which is all I thought motherhood was about back then. Nine years and three kids later, I realise that there are no 'answers'. Nor should there be, because motherhood is not a 'one-size-fits-all' experience. It's a constant work in progress. Every mum is unique. Every child is unique. The journey is your own.

So this book is not here to tell you what to do and why you should do it. It's here to give you a hug and make you laugh. To hold your hand when you're wondering if you're just making a sorry mess of the whole thing (you're not). To celebrate all the victories, no matter how small, and to allow you to remember, in years to come, just how brilliant and funny your preschooler was. Think of this book as that best friend who always says an empathetic or cheering word when you most need to hear it. Reassurance is the only guidance that has any real place or value, because you already have the other tools you need. Love and acceptance. You've had them from the moment you first held your baby in your arms and they will pretty much see you through, if you let them.

I hope *The Not-So-New Mum's Notebook* will help you feel good about yourself, and about how you're already raising your child(ren). I hope it will remind you that you're a 'good mum', just as you are. Because in the haze of raising human beings, it's so easy to lose sight of this. Motherhood is a calm blue sea one day and a raging stormy ocean the next. No matter how long we do it, we often feel a little like a fish out of water. It must be the only job where practice doesn't always make perfect because we're dealing with small human beings with beautiful minds of their own. The tide is always changing. As quickly as you get used to one stage, in a flash it's gone and you're cresting the wave of the next and clinging on for dear life.

> 66 What's there at the end of every joyful second, every frustrating moment and every neverending bedtime is unconditional love. 99

When we make our peace with the unpredictability of it all, when we relinquish the control we only ever really had in our minds, we allow ourselves to let go of the fear and panic that can be so debilitating – and instead enjoy the thrill of the ride. This happened to me, very naturally, when I had my third child. Unable to control anything to the degree that I once had, suddenly I was able to take a step back and just let stuff go. I was able to see what mattered (being happy in the moment right in front of us) and what didn't matter (everything else).

It has been the most liberating experience and has taken me to a calmer place in motherhood (albeit one where I still occasionally shout). Now, of all the things I doubt in my life, the way in which I'm raising my children is rarely one of them. I know, deep down in my core, that they are going to be ok. Not because I'm a perfect mum in any way, shape or form (she doesn't exist, by the way), but because what's there at the end of every joyful second, every frustrating moment and every neverending bedtime is unconditional love for my three wonderfully quirky kids.

Motherhood is the greatest project of our lives; the greatest privilege. Once we step over its threshold, we are never the same. We are stronger and more compassionate, without question.

Most importantly, we all do it differently and, as far as I can see, as long as we do it in a way that feels comfortable to us, with the company of other mums who get us, we're all going to be just fine. And so are our kids.

I believe this, wholeheartedly.

All my love to you,

Amy x

Motherhood.
the journey is
>your own.<

ON THIS DAY

DATE: _____

Be the mother you already are. Not the one you think you should be.

MY NOTES
(WHAT I LOVED, FELT, WISHED, NEEDED, STRUGGLED WITH, OVERCAME)

....

....

....

....

....

....

....

....

TO DO LIST

❑ ....

❑ ....

❑ ....

❑ ....

❑ ....

THINGS TO REMEMBER
(THAT I'LL PROBABLY STILL FORGET)

....

....

....

....

....

I'M ALREADY A GOOD MUM
(AND HERE'S A LIST OF REASONS WHY)

....

....

....

....

....

FUNNY THINGS YOU DID/SAID
(THANKS FOR MAKING ME LAUGH)

....

....

....

....

....

....

....

....

....

....

....

....

....

....

WHAT I WANT YOU TO KNOW
(YEARS FROM NOW)

....

....

....

....

....

....

....

....

....

....

....

....

....

Suddenly
she saw herself
through her child's eyes.
She told herself she
was a good mother.

And she set
herself free.

ON THIS DAY

DATE: _____

You already have everything you'll ever need. Your instincts.

MY NOTES
(WHAT I LOVED, FELT, WISHED, NEEDED, STRUGGLED WITH, OVERCAME)

....

....

....

....

....

....

....

....

....

....

....

TO DO LIST

❏ ....

❏ ....

❏ ....

❏ ....

❏ ....

YOU ARE A GREAT MUM
(JUST AS YOU ARE)

BE THE MOTHER YOU ALREADY ARE

It's very natural, in our roles as mothers, to try to constantly define, and then change, what sort of mother we are. We try on different 'mum' personas in a desperate attempt to figure out which one fits, without realising that we can be them all. Earth Mother. Routine Mother. Baking Mother. Calm Mother. Creative Mother. 'Trying to have it all' Mother. What we *should* be doing is accepting ourselves. The mother we already are. The mother who changes often because, first and foremost, she is a beautifully flawed chameleon of a woman. The mother who changes often because her child, environment and situation demands that she does. When my eldest was just a few months old, I wrote a list titled: 'The mother I want to be.' There were seventeen things on this list, including 'Be pro-active and decisive' and 'Put my children first but maintain a sense of self.' If I wrote it now there would probably be just one item – a mother who doesn't shout quite so much when the children fail to understand *again* what shoes are. But the thing is, I *am* a bit shouty. And whilst I used to waste a lot of time wishing I wasn't, I've made my peace with the fact that sometimes (especially when I'm frazzled) I am. It doesn't mean I can't *also* bake the occasional Victoria sponge, mess around with the children in the park, or sit calmly together with them and read a book. It just means that I don't need to be one thing or the other. I don't need to define the mother I am – or should be. I am already her.

BE A FLEXIBLE MOTHER

When my children were really small, I was continually advised to 'be consistent'. 'Whatever you do (and however badly you do it) consistency is key!' This is the message that surrounded me and the message that utterly overwhelmed me because I always found it *really* difficult to do. As my kids have grown, it feels even harder. Mainly because my kids still aren't consistent. And neither am I. Of course we're not. We're human beings. Individuals. To be consistent would assume that we exist in permanence. But we don't. I've lost count of the number of times I've felt rubbish because I haven't 'parented consistently'. I can see now that this is such a negative state of mind and all it does is set us up to fail. Because trying to be consistent all of the time, especially when you have more than one child, is blooming difficult, if not impossible. I have found that parenting flexibly works much better. It enables you to react to your kids in a responsive, rather than directive, way. It allows you to assess the situation at the very time that it is happening. To see that, today, your kids need an earlier night than last night. Because they are tired. Or that today they're going to eat dinner at the table, because you ate breakfast that morning on the sofa in front of the TV and they messed about. Parenting flexibly is about being in tune with your kids and yourself, not ploughing ahead despite them, on some pre-defined logic that doesn't take into account their changing needs, or yours, just because that's what you did last time. And the time before that. Parenting flexibly allows you to enjoy the natural ebb and flow of motherhood.

NEVER BEAT YOURSELF UP

Sometimes we parent in a way that doesn't feel comfortable. We lose our tempers. We raise our voices louder than we'd like. Afterwards, we feel awful. We feel that niggle at the pit of our stomach. We feel disappointed in ourselves and ashamed that our supermum self has let us down. Again. Damn her! When this happens, it's a signal for us to take notice, for us to learn from our reaction. But we should *never* beat ourselves up for it or expect that we'll never react that way again. Accept yourself, explain yourself to your child when you've calmed down, then move on. Because the moment has passed. Put your energies into creating a new, happier one. Kids do this very naturally, without any effort at all. They've long forgotten and forgiven, whilst we are still berating ourselves.

AS YOU ARE

You are a wonderful mother. As you are. So what if you play hide 'n' seek and hide just that little bit longer to get some 'me-time'? Or you once brushed your daughter's hair with a fork because you couldn't find the comb (true story). So what to any of it? Also, don't ever compare yourself to that mother who pops up on your social media feed. Who you allow to torment you because you perceive her to be so much more capable than you. She may have just done two hours of crafts but that is never the whole story. One minute we're throwing glue and glitter around with wild abandon, the next moment we're huffing and scooping peas off the floor. These ever-changing moments are the very nature of motherhood (and life). And we are all equal in it. As we are.

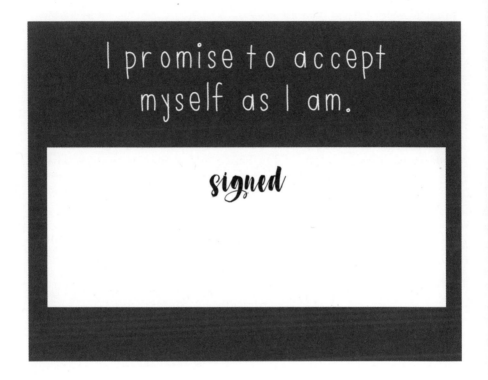

I promise to accept myself as I am.

signed

NO MUM GETS IT
RIGHT ALL OF
THE TIME. MOST OF US
ARE JUST FLYING
BY THE SEAT OF OUR
big comfy pants.

ON THIS DAY

DATE: _____

Never beat
yourself up.
Take note.
And move on.

MY NOTES
(WHAT I LOVED, FELT, WISHED, NEEDED, STRUGGLED WITH, OVERCAME)

....

....

....

....

....

....

....

....

TO DO LIST

❏ ....

❏ ....

❏ ....

❏ ....

❏ ....

THINGS TO REMEMBER
(THAT I'LL PROBABLY STILL FORGET)

....
....
....
....
....

THE MUM I THOUGHT I'D BE
(WRITE YOUR OWN 'SILLY' LIST)

....
....
....
....
....

FUNNY THINGS YOU DID/SAID
(THANKS FOR MAKING ME LAUGH)

....
....
....
....
....
....
....
....
....
....
....
....
....

WHAT I WANT YOU TO KNOW
(YEARS FROM NOW)

....
....
....
....
....
....
....
....
....
....
....
....
....

THERE ARE ALL
KINDS OF MUMS.
BE THE ONLY ONE
YOU CAN BE.
be you.

ON THIS DAY

DATE: _____

Mother like no one's watching. Because yours is the only opinion that matters.

MY NOTES
(WHAT I LOVED, FELT, WISHED, NEEDED, STRUGGLED WITH, OVERCAME)

....

....

....

....

....

....

....

....

....

....

....

TO DO LIST

❑ ....

❑ ....

❑ ....

❑ ....

❑ ....

WELCOME TO THE WONDERFUL, CRAZY WORLD OF TODDLERS

TODDLERS ARE SOMETHING ELSE

So. Now we've established that you're a great mum just as you are (don't worry, there are lots of reminders to come, for when you forget), let's talk about those delightful little beings that stop you from ever fulfilling your true potential as the 'Perfect Mother' (you see, it's not your fault). Toddlers. About now, you might be wondering where your sweet obliging baby went and who this slightly stroppy human is, bouncing frantically up and down in front of you (or on you) like Tigger. Toddlers are something else altogether. I have had three of them and I have NEVER been prepared for the frequent insaneness of them (whilst they are also simultaneously brilliant and captivating). Their very nature defies all logic, as they strive towards independence. Theirs, I should add. Not yours. No, your independence is about to be shot to s*** even more, as you are forced to follow your newly toddling toddler everywhere and police every crazy thing they want to do. And my, is it crazy.

PLAYING WITH ANYTHING THAT ISN'T A TOY

Cake tins. Dried pulses and other choking hazards. Your online banking thingy. It doesn't really matter. The only thing you need to know here is that traditional toys suck. Toddlers have no interest in anything safe or age-appropriate, even if it's brightly coloured, plastic and would have flashing lights (had you been able to find any batteries and unscrew that annoying flap on the bottom). Quite frankly, you're insulting their intelligence by even getting these out. Save your money and spend it on a nice lipstick instead. (Oh and don't get all clever and go and buy a toy online banking thingy because they like yours so much and John Lewis do a really cute pretend one. Toddlers can smell a fake a mile off.)

THE SINK

Opening the cupboard door under the sink. Repeatedly. No one has ever shown them this chasm. Yet from the moment they can move, somehow they know it exists. Yes, your toddler who won't so much as touch a floret of organic broccoli will have an overwhelming penchant for Mr Muscle.

WANTING STUFF THEY CAN'T HAVE

If I had to sum up a toddler's agenda in one sentence, I would probably say this: 'I want the only thing you won't let me have.' You could have a room FULL of everything they usually like. The online banking thingy. Your purse with all those lovely plastic cards that you totally don't need, until you're at the checkout and can't find any of them (don't worry, your toddler has safely 'stored' them down the side of the sofa. You'll never find them, of course, because, erm, you haven't hoovered under the sofa cushions since circa 2003). No, if there is one thing in that room that you don't want them to have, not only will they find it, but when you tell them they can't have it, they will lose the will to live. And then, so will you.

ANYTHING REMOTELY DANGEROUS

This excludes pretty much nothing, because if a thing isn't already dangerous, toddlers will find a way to make it so. I mean, why go down a slide when you can walk up it and risk getting booted in the head by another child playing by the rules? It's an actual miracle they make it to the preschool years. Eventually, you will have to pile EVERYTHING you own up high, where you can never reach it again. You might as well just chuck it all away now.

GOING UP THE STAIRS. AND BACK DOWN AGAIN

Buy a stair gate. Don't buy a stair gate. It's irrelevant. Because at some point they are going to discover stairs. And at some point you are going to spend your entire day discovering stairs, too. For about a year. Putting up a barrier might just make them more desirable. Probably best to just suck it up and get it over and done with now. Like most things in parenting.

FOLLOWING YOU AROUND

Toddlers aren't great at keeping their own company. And they don't much like other toddlers. So they want your company. For every waking minute of every single day. So you can do all the fun stuff together. Like going up the stairs. And back down again.

SNOTTY KISSES

To the rest of the world, that slightly grubby face with a snotty nose (from all the tantrums and crying) is pretty repulsive. Yuk. But when those chubby arms grab the back of your neck and your toddler leans in for a proper, snotty smooch, that's pretty much love, right there. And it sort of (totally) makes up for all the 'trying to kill themselves' (and you) stuff.

today I loved my toddler because...

....

....

....

....

....

toddler (n.)

Never toddles.
Hurtles towards things -
always in the opposite
direction to you.
Creates havoc. And tries
to kill themselves 1,372
times a day.

ON THIS DAY

DATE: _____

If you sometimes feel like you're losing your mind, it's only temporary. Promise.

MY NOTES
(WHAT I LOVED, FELT, WISHED, NEEDED, STRUGGLED WITH, OVERCAME)

....

....

....

....

....

....

....

....

....

....

....

....

TO DO LIST

❏ ....

❏ ....

❏ ....

❏ ....

❏ ....

THINGS TO REMEMBER
(THAT I'LL PROBABLY STILL FORGET)

....
....
....
....
....

HOW YOU DROVE ME MAD
(WAYS YOU TRIED TO KILL YOURSELF TODAY)

....
....
....
....
....

FUNNY THINGS YOU DID/SAID
(THANKS FOR MAKING ME LAUGH)

....
....
....
....
....
....
....
....
....
....
....
....
....
....

WHAT I WANT YOU TO KNOW
(YEARS FROM NOW)

....
....
....
....
....
....
....
....
....
....
....
....
....
....

TODDLERS CAN MAKE
TWELVE HOURS
FEEL LIKE TWENTY-FOUR.
TAKE A *breather*
WHEN YOU CAN.
HIDE IN THE BATHROOM.

(No judgement.)

ON THIS DAY

DATE: _____

Sometimes there's no reasoning with a toddler. Like everything, THIS WILL PASS.

MY NOTES
(WHAT I LOVED, FELT, WISHED, NEEDED, STRUGGLED WITH, OVERCAME)

....

....

....

....

....

....

....

....

TO DO LIST

☐ ....

....

☐ ....

....

☐ ....

....

☐ ....

....

☐ ....

SLEEP, BEDHOPPING AND OTHER STALLING TECHNIQUES

SLEEP IS THE NEW SEX

Many mums with sleepless children are surprised (and understandably disappointed) when they discover that their baby growing older doesn't necessarily mean they miraculously start sleeping. For all the toddlers who are 'obediently' going to bed at 7.00 pm and rising at 7.00 am, there are many, many more doing their own merry thing: refusing to go to bed; getting up several times once they're there; waking habitually at 5.00 am, keen to start their day (even though absolutely no one else is). Sleep is our biggest obsession as parents. Lack of it. Desire for it. Fantasising about it. It's the equivalent of those conversations with your friends, where you used to talk about how much sex you were (or weren't) having. 'I got eight hours sleep last night,' says someone. Gasps all round.

'THAT IS NOT MY BEDROOM!'

But the fact is, no matter how well you 'train' your child, their sleep habits will almost constantly change – just like your child. So many things can throw it off course. Illness, particularly coughs, colds and snotty noses, which can make sleep almost impossible. Developmental phases, such as your child becoming more mobile and doing an Alcatraz-style escape out of their cot, forcing you to take the sides down AGAINST YOUR WILL (this type of milestone is never a joyous one). Teething (if in doubt, blame teething). Ironically, I think my sleep has actually got worse as my kids have got older (sorry to say this out loud). Having raised two Gina Ford girls with a routine so strict you'd have wondered if Gina was watching (and one Gerry Ford, who did his own wonderfully random thing), my daughters slept fairly well and consistently when they were babies. Now that they are older, we have all manner of bedtime disruptions from all three of them. 'Just one more Netflix episode PLEASE!' (repeated 362 times). 'But we haven't had dinner!' (they have). And my absolute favourite from my then two-year-old, 'That is NOT my bedroom!' (Like, seriously, are you blooming kidding me?)

THE JOYS OF BEDHOPPING

Remember when your mum told you 'nice girls don't sleep around?' Well, there have been mornings where I have woken up with NO IDEA where I am or how I got there. There were a couple of years in our house, when the three kids spanned one to six years old, where bedhopping was almost a nightly pursuit. So much fun! 'Let's all go to sleep and see how many beds we can sleep in/not sleep in/ditch in favour of someone else's that's so much more comfortable.' I'm telling you, Goldilocks had nothing on us. Even now, one of my kids usually sneaks in and nuzzles up next to me at some point in the small hours. And there are weeks where I think I probably manage only one night a week with NO ONE ELSE in my bed. It goes against everything Gina told me to do, but it doesn't make me unhappy or stressed anymore. I don't lose sleep over it (pardon the metaphor, because I obviously do). I don't catastrophise it. I don't imagine that my kids will still be doing this shizzle when they're eighteen. Because they won't, will they? They'll be out, beyond curfew, and I still won't be getting any sleep worrying about where they are. In summary: do what you need to do and don't beat yourself up about it. Let them sleep with you. Don't let them sleep with you. Do a mixture of both. Know your limits and go about implementing a strategy when you're utterly broken and JUST NEED SLEEP, even if this means giving the kid(s) to a family member overnight or you going to bed by 8.00 pm. Whatever you do, DON'T PANIC. Sleep is not really ours for the taking like it was before we became parents. And when we get on board with this, we somehow feel more comfortable about it and realise that it's just how it is, for now. One day, some glorious moment in the future, our sleep will once again be under our own control. Till then, do what works.

HELPING YOURSELF

My dear gran always used to say that the most important sleeping hours were the two hours before midnight. She was absolutely right and, on the rare occasions when I do get to bed by 10.00 pm, I have always noticed the difference the next day, even if I've been disturbed during the night. What us parents are brilliant at doing is going to bed ridiculously late, despite being shattered. That need for some kid-free time means we don't help ourselves. Kid-free time is important, but try to alternate and get to bed early every other night, so you keep your sleep reserves (sort of) topped up. I'll do it if you will.

TRICK YOUR MIND INTO GETTING MORE SLEEP

There is a saving grace. And it is this: we can teach ourselves to think about sleep differently. Eight hours be the holy grail, but if that's not realistic (and for so many parents it obviously isn't), don't start your day off counting how many hours you've had (or not had). Cognitive Behavioural Therapy (CBT), a talking therapy that can help you manage your problems by changing the way you think and behave, teaches us that this is a really unhelpful practice. It just makes us focus on lack and sends us spiralling into a place where all we can think about is how tired we are. Far better to get up, shower, have a nice cup of tea or pop an energy tablet into a pint of water, grab some breakfast and live the day ahead, whether it's one that might allow a sneaky afternoon nap or a full-on day at work with lots of coffee and a barrel of biscuits.

Sleep, like most things is in the eye of the beholder. You can choose to change how you see it.

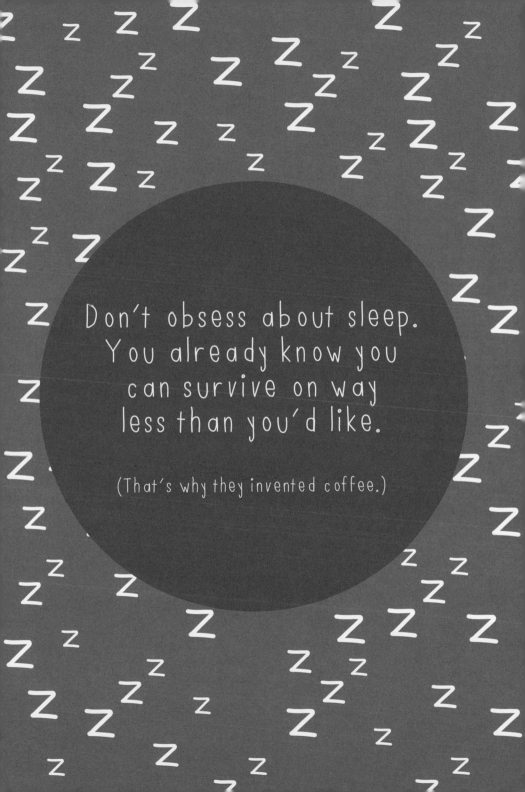

Don't obsess about sleep.
You already know you
can survive on way
less than you'd like.

(That's why they invented coffee.)

ON THIS DAY

DATE: _____

Go to bed at 10.00 pm and get those precious two pre-midnight hours.

MY NOTES
(WHAT I LOVED, FELT, WISHED, NEEDED, STRUGGLED WITH, OVERCAME)

....

....

....

....

....

....

....

....

....

....

....

TO DO LIST

☐ ....

☐ ....

☐ ....

☐ ....

☐ ....

THINGS TO REMEMBER
(THAT I'LL PROBABLY STILL FORGET)

....

....

....

....

....

WHEN I'M SLEEP DEPRIVED
(THINGS THAT HELP ME FEEL BETTER)

....

....

....

....

....

FUNNY THINGS YOU DID/SAID
(THANKS FOR MAKING ME LAUGH)

....

....

....

....

....

....

....

....

....

....

....

....

....

WHAT I WANT YOU TO KNOW
(YEARS FROM NOW)

....

....

....

....

....

....

....

....

....

....

....

....

....

THERE ARE NO MIRACLES
TO GET KIDS TO SLEEP.
AND TO STAY IN THEIR BEDS.
SO DO WHATEVER
YOU NEED TO DO.
WHATEVER WORKS.
AND *never panic.*

(They won't be doing it when
they're eighteen, promise.)

ON THIS DAY

DATE: _____

Daytime naps aren't just for new mums. Go on. Treat yourself.

MY NOTES
(WHAT I LOVED, FELT, WISHED, NEEDED, STRUGGLED WITH, OVERCAME)

....

....

....

....

....

....

....

....

....

....

....

TO DO LIST

❏ ....

❏ ....

❏ ....

❏ ....

❏ ....

THE NOT-SO-NEW MUM'S POWER BREAKFAST

When you've had a bad night's sleep (or no sleep at all), it's so easy to, a) miss breakfast altogether; b) reach for the biscuits; or c) drink ALL the coffee on an empty stomach and give yourself the jitters. I never missed breakfast until I had kids and found myself far too busy seeing to their needs. The thing is, this only ends one way – with you feeling even worse. So, do yourself a favour, occupy your child with some television or a colouring book for fifteen minutes and cook yourself this. It will regulate the blood sugar and stop you craving what we all want when we're tired: SUGAR. The protein from the eggs, mushrooms and peanut butter will satisfy your hunger, whilst that superfood, spinach, is high in everything, including magnesium, which is great for calming anxiety and good for neurological function. The density of rye bread can take some getting used to, but it's a great alternative to its wheat counterparts, retaining more nutrients and making you feel less bloated afterwards.

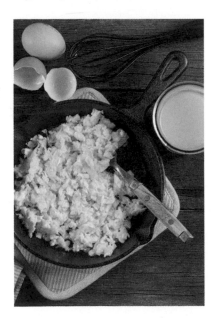

INGREDIENTS

5 or 6 mushrooms, cut into quarters

Butter or olive oil, for frying

3 eggs

2 slices of rye bread

1 tablespoon of peanut butter

Good handful of washed, raw spinach

METHOD

Fry or grill the mushrooms in a little butter or olive oil in a frying pan over a high heat to get them lovely and brown. At the same time, crack the eggs into a hot saucepan, whisk with a fork and cook on a low heat, stirring often as you scramble them.

Toast the rye bread and spread one slice with butter and the other with peanut butter. Remove the eggs from the heat whilst they are still moist and stir in a small knob of butter, and season with salt and pepper. Top the buttered rye bread with the eggs, raw spinach (which will wilt from the heat) and the mushrooms. Serve the peanut butter rye bread on the side, dig in and feel better.

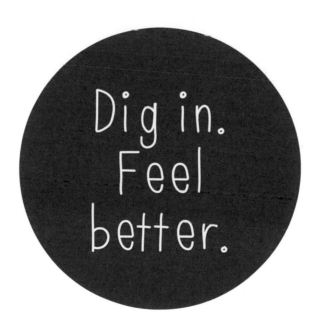

ON THIS DAY

DATE: _____

Nurture your body with some proper food every once in a while. MAKE TIME.

MY NOTES
(WHAT I LOVED, FELT, WISHED, NEEDED, STRUGGLED WITH, OVERCAME)

....

....

....

....

....

....

....

....

....

....

....

....

TO DO LIST

❏ ....

❏ ....

❏ ....

❏ ....

❏ ....

THINGS TO REMEMBER
(THAT I'LL PROBABLY STILL FORGET)

....
....
....
....
....

FOODS THAT FUEL ME
(HEALTHY SNACKS I LIKE)

....
....
....
....
....

FUNNY THINGS YOU DID/SAID
(THANKS FOR MAKING ME LAUGH)

....
....
....
....
....
....
....
....
....
....
....
....
....

WHAT I WANT YOU TO KNOW
(YEARS FROM NOW)

....
....
....
....
....
....
....
....
....
....
....
....
....

45

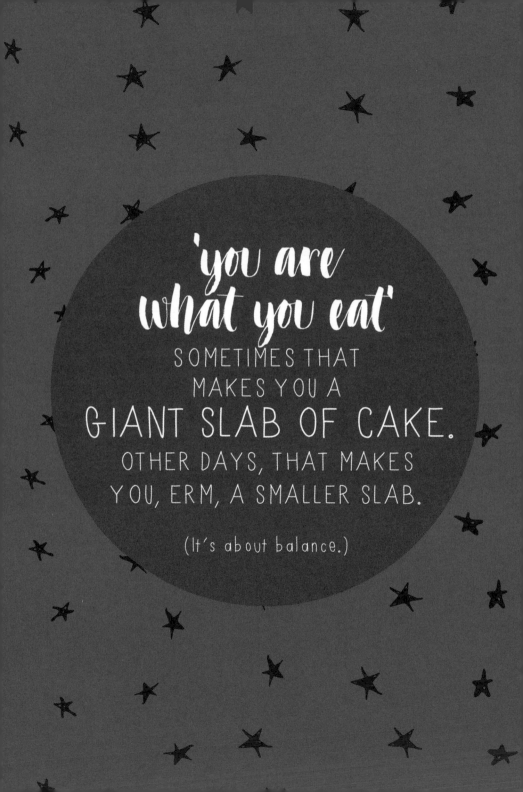

'you are what you eat'
SOMETIMES THAT MAKES YOU A GIANT SLAB OF CAKE. OTHER DAYS, THAT MAKES YOU, ERM, A SMALLER SLAB.

(It's about balance.)

ON THIS DAY

DATE: _____

Can't beat that sugar craving? Get your hands on some protein.

MY NOTES
(WHAT I LOVED, FELT, WISHED, NEEDED, STRUGGLED WITH, OVERCAME)

....

....

....

....

....

....

TO DO LIST

☐ ....

☐ ....

☐ ....

☐ ....

☐ ....

DOING STUFF WITH WILFUL TODDLERS (AND INSTANTLY REGRETTING IT)

Attempting activities with strong-minded toddlers who move and have opinions can be different to doing stuff with a buggy-obliging baby. You may already be realising this. Here are some things you might want to avoid. (If you have a toddler who's pretty chilled, you can just read this, thank your lucky stars and enjoy the entertainment value because *obviously* I'm exaggerating. Or am I?)

EATING OUT WITH KIDS

Who doesn't like eating out with toddlers? (Ok, those with calm ones might.) The adrenaline rush of it all. What will they throw? How long will they sit still? Will they actually eat anything or will you hand over a fiver for a 'happy' meal that could be happier? I have this whole joyful experience down to a fine art now. Firstly, conduct a full risk assessment as soon as you enter the restaurant. Make a note of all available exits, glasses, knives and stairs. There will always be something you miss. But don't worry, your toddler will spot it long before you. Apologise to the waiting staff in advance so they're slightly more sympathetic when your toddler throws a dough ball at them. Or a fork. Apologise to other diners in advance. For the same reason. Don't waste money ordering actual food for your toddler. Toddlers don't eat, remember? Unless it's a bowl of lollipops. Drink wine (you). In fact, forget the food and just order wine. A bottle (no glass). It's easier to consume than a bowl of pasta whilst running after a toddler on the rampage. Pay your bill. When your toddler's having a full on meltdown because you won't let them decapitate themselves with the stray knife you missed (killjoy), it's easy to forget basic manners like, erm, paying for what you've had. But the fact is, after exposing everyone else in the restaurant to your 'spirited' toddler, you should probably be paying bills as well as yours. My top tip? Don't eat out. Ever. Stay at home. Serve up £1.99 fish fingers. And let your toddler throw those around instead. It's way cheaper. And just as much fun.

GOING TO THE CINEMA

If you went to baby cinema you'll have lovely, nostalgic memories of how good that was. Then one day you'll think, 'Oh, I know. Let's go and see that new Disney film. That will be nice.' No. That won't be nice. Because your 'baby' is now a mobile toddler. And they don't much like sitting still. So you'll spend the entire film following them up and down the aisle steps on your hands and knees, whilst eyeing up your (now cold) bacon butty and latte.

SHOPPING

Two words. The internet. This is basically why it was invented. So parents could buy stuff. Going to the supermarket (or any shop, come to that) with a toddler and expecting to actually come back with something you can make a meal out of is optimistic, at best. Ironically, I didn't start trying to do my shopping in an actual supermarket again until my third toddler, after I kept falling asleep during the online shop and then had to figure out how to make a lamb tagine with sixteen Twix bars and a can of chickpeas. 'I'll go to the shops!' I thought in one of my light-bulb that-will-come-back-to-bite-me-on-the-a*** moments. Lo and behold, it was a disaster. After begging/forcing/bribing said toddler to get into the trolley, every time my back was turned, he touched something, licked it, ate it. When we got to the checkout, he managed to reach and press a random button on the till and brought the entire supermarket's computer system to a halt. Think Y2K, but with sticky hands. It took twenty minutes to reboot. Suffice to say, we now enjoy Twix Tagine at least once a week.

EVERYTHING ELSE

Basically, anything that I haven't covered above. You can do stuff again when they go to school. If you can be bothered by then.

ON THIS DAY

Take the easy option whenever you can. And conserve your energy.

DATE: _____

MY NOTES
(WHAT I LOVED, FELT, WISHED, NEEDED, STRUGGLED WITH, OVERCAME)

....
....
....
....
....
....
....
....
....
....

TO DO LIST

☐ ....
☐ ....
☐ ....
☐ ....
☐ ....

THINGS TO REMEMBER
(THAT I'LL PROBABLY STILL FORGET)

....

....

....

....

....

TODDLER-SAFE ACTIVITIES
(LIST OF PLAYGROUPS, CLASSES, SOFT PLAY)

....

....

....

....

....

FUNNY THINGS YOU DID/SAID
(THANKS FOR MAKING ME LAUGH)

....

....

....

....

....

....

....

....

....

....

....

....

....

WHAT I WANT YOU TO KNOW
(YEARS FROM NOW)

....

....

....

....

....

....

....

....

....

....

....

....

....

The **simple things** won't always feel so **challenging.** So embrace this time and use the opportunity to keep life **slow.**

(You'll be rushing soon enough when they start school.)

ON THIS DAY

DATE: _____

It's ok to lose your temper through frustration or tiredness. Some days are hard.

MY NOTES
(WHAT I LOVED, FELT, WISHED, NEEDED, STRUGGLED WITH, OVERCAME)

....

....

....

....

....

....

....

....

....

....

....

TO DO LIST

❏ ....

❏ ....

❏ ....

❏ ....

❏ ....

SOME KIDS ONLY EAT BEIGE FOOD (AND THAT'S OK)

FOOD, GLORIOUS FOOD!

Mealtime – the time when mums are most likely to be found pulling their hair out. Feeding young kids can be stressful, unrewarding and really hard to master. Despite everyone telling you not to worry when your child isn't eating or they refuse to exist on anything other than plain pasta or a beige banquet from the freezer, it physically hurts that nurturing bit of your heart and soul. It doesn't matter how many inventive ways you find to hide vegetables in a sauce, your toddler just knows. Their sixth sense has picked up that you are trying to trick them with SOMETHING THAT IS NOT BEIGE. Well, would you mind if I tell you NOT to worry? That it's all going to be ok and your toddler is NOT always going to eat like this. That one day, they *may* even voluntarily eat a bit of cabbage or spinach? I am not kidding.

THERE IS A REASON FOR FUSSY EATING

Somewhere along this merry journey of feeding my kids, I learned about food neophobia, which occurs in children at around 18 months to two years old. Apparently, it's an evolutionary trait designed to protect them from harm, which results in them treating anything new with suspicion, presumably dating back to more primitive times when they were much more likely to be exposed to red berries and wild mushrooms that could literally kill them. It doesn't matter if this seems a bit far-fetched now, when you're serving them a completely sterile chicken casserole. Don't you feel just a little bit better for having a rational reason for their pickiness?

HOW TO GET YOUR KID(S) TO EAT

Put it on your plate and look like you're enjoying it. This method is almost foolproof. I can serve identical foods on different plates. Theirs will be pushed aside in disgust and, seconds later, they'll be tucking into mine and saying, 'Mmmmmmm'. Other tactics include eliminating snacks – fussy kids are *much* more likely to eat when they're really hungry – and serving what you know they'll eat, even if they *have* had it five days in a row. This will save your sanity, if nothing else and it won't do them any harm. For about two years, my middle child would only eat plain pasta with butter. Sometimes, she'd be *really* wild and have a bagel. It used to kill me. At the age of six, she now scoffs down a full roast dinner; broccoli, carrots and all. What's better, her four-year-old brother, who pretty much weaned himself on chocolate fingers and anything he found on the car floor, copies her (one perk of having multiple children). Finally, you can always offset all the beige stuff and get some actual nutrients down them with one of those fruit or vegetable pouches you buy during weaning, even if they're WAY past the weaning stage. It doesn't matter how you do it; just find a way that works for you.

DITCH THE NUTRITIONAL GUILT

Probably the most unhelpful thing we do as mums, first-time ones especially, is completely obsess over this eating lark. It's understandable; we want them to be healthy, grow strong and develop good eating habits. But putting so much pressure on ourselves and them isn't good for anyone. Kids pick up on our anxiety, our well-meaning tendency to over-parent, and they respond accordingly. Having three kids has shown me this over and over again in every aspect of motherhood, from eating habits to potty training. The third child really *has* raised himself, and done it far better than me. So when it comes to dinnertime and the chips are down/burned/all over the floor, know one thing and remind yourself of it often: do whatever works, ditch the guilt and trust that it won't always be like this (ok, that's three things). This mantra applies to pretty much everything in parenthood.

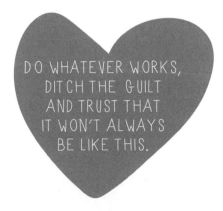

DO WHATEVER WORKS, DITCH THE GUILT AND TRUST THAT IT WON'T ALWAYS BE LIKE THIS.

ON THIS DAY

DATE: _____

If you're fed up of feeding dinner to the bin, just serve something you know your child will eat.

MY NOTES
(WHAT I LOVED, FELT, WISHED, NEEDED, STRUGGLED WITH, OVERCAME)

....

....

....

....

....

....

....

....

....

....

....

TO DO LIST

❏ ....

❏ ....

❏ ....

❏ ....

❏ ....

THINGS TO REMEMBER
(THAT I'LL PROBABLY STILL FORGET)

....

....

....

....

....

FOODS YOU LIKE/DISLIKE
(SO YOU ACTUALLY EAT SOMETHING)

....

....

....

....

....

FUNNY THINGS YOU DID/SAID
(THANKS FOR MAKING ME LAUGH)

....

....

....

....

....

....

....

....

....

....

....

....

WHAT I WANT YOU TO KNOW
(YEARS FROM NOW)

....

....

....

....

....

....

....

....

....

....

....

....

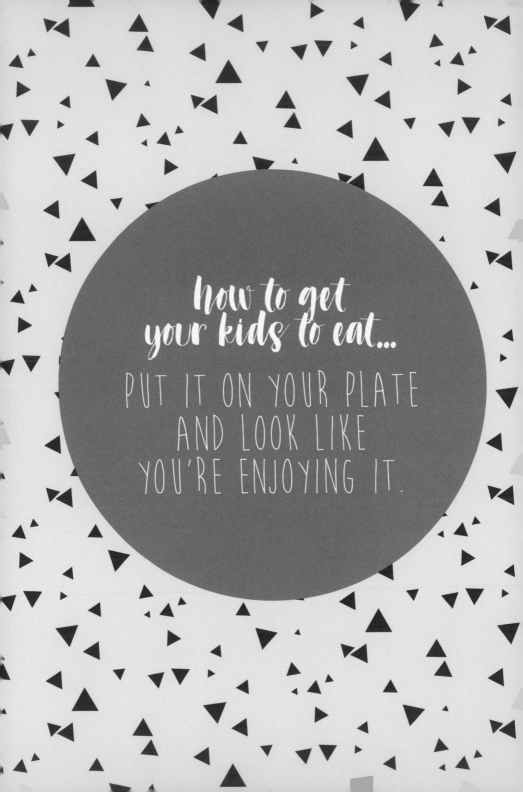

how to get
your kids to eat...
PUT IT ON YOUR PLATE
AND LOOK LIKE
YOU'RE ENJOYING IT.

ON THIS DAY

DATE: _____

MY NOTES
(WHAT I LOVED, FELT, WISHED, NFFDED, STRUGGLED WITH, OVERCAME)

....

....

....

....

....

....

....

....

....

....

....

TO DO LIST

☐ ....

☐ ....

☐ ....

☐ ....

☐ ....

'WHAT MUMS SAY TO GET US TO EAT' (BY A TWO-YEAR-OLD)

Mums. They're weird about this eating business. When it comes to me NOT eating my dinner, she gets, well, a bit mad. Nothing else bothers her as much as me not eating. My friends say their mums are the same. We don't get their obsession with it, we really don't. This is just SOME of the stuff my mum says when I'm flinging my spoon everywhere and decorating the floor/walls/cat.

1. 'Children in Africa would love to be eating your dinner.'
This is her favourite line. She says it a lot. I have no idea what she's talking about. Where is Africa anyway? And if I'm not eating my dinner then surely it's a good thing because anything I don't eat can go to those other kids in Africa? Wherever that is.

2. 'If you don't eat your dinner, you're not having a yoghurt.'
So what? I don't even like yoghurts anymore. At least tempt me with something I WANT to eat. Like chocolate ice cream. I know you'll never give me that anyway so there's absolutely no incentive to eat my dinner here. None whatsoever. Sorry.

3. 'You liked peas yesterday...?'
Well today I don't. I've gone right off them. I actually fancy some tomatoes. What do you mean you didn't think I liked tomatoes? Today, I DO like tomatoes actually.

4. 'Just five more mouthfuls and then you can have a yoghurt...'
Ahh the yoghurt bribe again. When will you realise that yoghurts just don't float my boat? I quite enjoy this debate though, because I always manage to negotiate her down to three more mouthfuls. Then I spit one of those on the floor when she's not looking.

5. 'If you don't eat, you won't grow up to be big and strong.'
Big and strong in comparison to who? The Incredible Hulk? Because honestly, I don't really want to look like him. If that's ok with you. So I'll carry on eating like a sparrow.

6. 'The TV's going off if you don't start eating.'
I'm a bit confused by this one. One of the house rules is no TV on when I'm eating. So why it's on in the first place is a mystery. But I'm not going to point this out. Obviously.

7. 'I've worked really hard preparing this food for you. Some children don't even get home-cooked dinners.'
Oh no, she's going to start talking about Africa again. Any. Minute. Now. I'm not sure what she means by 'really hard'. Is putting some pasta in a pan with some frozen vegetables that difficult? Then sieving it and throwing in a bit of cream cheese. It's not exactly Gordon Ramsay is it? Yes, I've seen the cooking programmes...
I know what I'm missing.

8. 'Right, that's it, I'm not cooking any more. You can just eat cakes and rubbish.'
Finally. We're getting somewhere. She understands. This is exactly what I WANT to eat. Sadly, I know she'll never keep to her word. And tomorrow we'll be going through the whole shebang again.

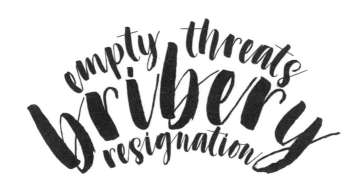

61

ON THIS DAY

DATE: _____

It doesn't matter if your child eats the same thing day in, day out. They will grow out of it.

MY NOTES
(WHAT I LOVED, FELT, WISHED, NEEDED, STRUGGLED WITH, OVERCAME)

....
....
....
....
....
....
....
....

TO DO LIST

❏ ....
❏ ....
❏ ....
❏ ....
❏ ....

THINGS TO REMEMBER
(THAT I'LL PROBABLY STILL FORGET)

....
....
....
....
....

FAILSAFE RECIPES
(THAT YOU'LL PROBABLY GO OFF)

....
....
....
....
....

FUNNY THINGS YOU DID/SAID
(THANKS FOR MAKING ME LAUGH)

....
....
....
....
....
....
....
....
....
....
....
....

WHAT I WANT YOU TO KNOW
(YEARS FROM NOW)

....
....
....
....
....
....
....
....
....
....
....
....

WHEN IT COMES TO
SMALL KIDS AND FOOD?

beige is the new black.

(which means you're bang on trend.)

ON THIS DAY

DATE: _____

Cut down your child's snacks. It's amazing what they'll eat when they're really hungry.

MY NOTES
(WHAT I LOVED, FELT, WISHED, NEEDED, STRUGGLED WITH, OVERCAME)

....

....

....

....

....

....

....

....

....

....

....

TO DO LIST

❏ ....

❏ ....

❏ ....

❏ ....

❏ ....

10-MINUTE RECIPES YOUR CHILD WILL (HOPEFULLY) EAT

Here are a few tried-and-tested recipes that my three kids (usually) eat and even enjoy. They're quick, easy and are made with stuff you're likely to have in your kitchen. Each recipe serves one. Simply multiply the ingredients accordingly if you want to serve additional kids/yourself and a partner or freeze some for later.

POPEYE PASTA

A very green dish that my kids have always, surprisingly, loved.
Popeye's favourite.

50g pasta
Knob of butter
1/4 bag spinach, washed
1 tablespoon cream cheese
Splash of milk
*Sauce is freezable. Defrost before use.

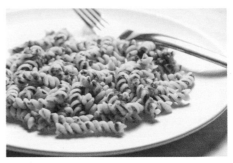

Cook the pasta as per the packet instructions. In another pan, melt the butter on a low heat, add the spinach and cook until wilted. Squeeze and drain the spinach with the back of a spoon, pouring out any excess liquid, then add the cream cheese and milk and stir. Puree with a handheld blender until smooth, then mix in the pasta and serve.

STICKY HONEY CHICKEN

1 chicken thigh (skinless and boneless)
Small glug of olive oil
Drizzle of honey
Carrots/sweet potato/any veg
that can be glazed

Turn on your oven and heat to 180°C/* Gas Mark 4. Put the chicken in a small ovenproof dish. Drizzle with the olive oil and honey and stir until covered. Add the vegetables and coat with the glaze. Bake in the oven for 25 minutes, turning over halfway through. Make sure the chicken is cooked through before serving.

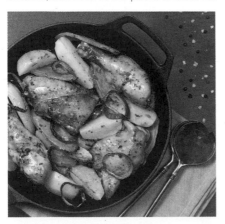

EGG-FRIED RICE

50g rice
2 tablespoons peas/sweetcorn/frozen
vegetables
Small glug of olive oil
1 egg
*Not freezable/reheatable

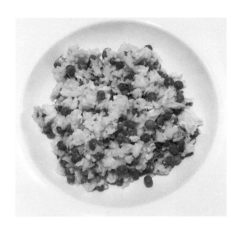

Cook the rice in a pan of boiling water for 6 minutes. Add whatever frozen veg you're using and cook for a further 5 minutes. Drain and put back in the pan. Make a well in the centre, heat the olive oil, crack the egg in and stir it, drawing the rice into it. Cook for a couple of minutes until the egg is set and serve.

TEATIME MEZZE

Basically, you call it a 'mezze' and feel better about serving up a cold tea. Win win, right? Here are some ideas for what you might include:

Oatcakes/breadsticks/crackers/
Twiglets/anything beige...
Dollop of ready-made houmous/
mashed avocado
Cucumber/carrot sticks
Tomatoes (halved or quartered)
Cubes of cheese/pre-cooked chicken
chunks/slices of cooked meat
Boiled egg, quartered
Olives (wash off the brine if they've
been sitting in salty water)
Raisins/blueberries/grapes (halve
grapes lengthways)
Sliced apple/satsuma pieces/pear
quarters

Serve a selection in portions on a plate and let them get messy! Or use a muffin tin for each different food type to ramp up the 'fun' factor. This is a great way to encourage them to try new things.

MEATBALL METEORS

A quick alternative to bolognese. Tell the kids they've just landed from space...
As a great way of using up leftovers, you can include any of their favourite vegetables you have knocking around – the ones mentioned below are just for inspiration.

50g pasta/rice
Small glug of olive oil
3 ready prepared meatballs
(or beef/lamb/turkey/pork mince
rolled into little balls)
Optional carrots, peppers or
mushrooms, cut up into small pieces
100ml passata/chopped tomatoes
Squirt of tomato ketchup
*Sauce and meatballs are freezable. Defrost before use. Never reheat rice.

Cook the pasta or rice as per the packet instructions. Heat the olive oil in a frying pan, add the meatballs and cook until browned. Fry the vegetables in the same pan, if you're using them. Add the passata or tomatoes and a good squirt of tomato ketchup to sweeten the sauce. Simmer on a low heat for 10 minutes until cooked through. Stir in the pasta/rice and serve.

Even the fussiest of kids are eating a wide range of foods by the time they hit school age. It's going to be ok. **Promise.**

ON THIS DAY

DATE: _____

Maybe your child just doesn't feel like eating. Try again later.

MY NOTES
(WHAT I LOVED, FELT, WISHED, NEEDED, STRUGGLED WITH, OVERCAME)

....

....

....

....

....

....

....

....

....

....

....

TO DO LIST

☐ ....

☐ ....

☐ ....

☐ ....

☐ ....

ON THIS DAY

DATE: _____

Serving up
a kid's
ready meal
won't kill
them. FACT.

MY NOTES
(WHAT I LOVED, FELT, WISHED, NEEDED, STRUGGLED WITH, OVERCAME)

....

....

....

....

....

....

....

....

....

....

....

TO DO LIST

❏ ....

❏ ....

❏ ....

❏ ....

❏ ....

THINGS TO REMEMBER
(THAT I'LL PROBABLY STILL FORGET)

....

....

....

....

....

QUICK MEALS FOR ME
(HEALTHY RECIPES WITHOUT FUSS)

....

....

....

....

....

FUNNY THINGS YOU DID/SAID
(THANKS FOR MAKING ME LAUGH)

....

....

....

....

....

....

....

....

....

....

....

....

....

....

WHAT I WANT YOU TO KNOW
(YEARS FROM NOW)

....

....

....

....

....

....

....

....

....

....

....

....

....

....

They'll eat poo
from the garden.
A crust they've found under
a park bench. But that 'slop'
you made from scratch?
You're having a laugh,
aren't you?

ON THIS DAY

DATE: _____

Don't compare your child's eating habits to someone else's. ALL kids go through phases.

MY NOTES
(WHAT I LOVED, FELT, WISHED, NEEDED, STRUGGLED WITH, OVERCAME)

....

....

....

....

....

....

....

....

....

....

....

TO DO LIST

❑ ....

❑ ....

❑ ....

❑ ....

❑ ....

73

HELL HATH NO FURY LIKE A TODDLER

'WHY ARE YOU RUINING MY LIFE?'

If toddlers could actually verbalise what it is they're feeling, is what they would say: 'WHY ARE YOU RUINING MY LIFE?' Because toddlers are really easy to p*** off. Like, easy. You've probably noticed you can pretty much do it without even trying, most days. It's quite a skill. The fact that you're not intentionally making them angry is beside the point. And how you talk them down from the height of their rage is something else altogether.

THINGS THAT ANNOY TODDLERS

So far, from personal experience, I have discovered that the following things annoy toddlers:

1. Serving their porridge too hot. Serving it too cold. Serving it at all.
2. Making clothes choices for them based on the weather or anything remotely logical. There must be a reason why they want to wear sweaty, rubbery wellies in summer and sandals in winter. I haven't found it yet, but what do I know?
3. Stopping them from killing themselves by playing in the road, climbing a ladder or amputating limbs/fingers in doors. None of which they've ever thanked me for. I'm just that irritating woman who ruins all their fun.
4. Giving their dinner – which they didn't want – to the bin/dog/a sibling. At which point it becomes highly desirable and the only thing they can think about.
5. Asking them to have a bath. Telling them they can't have a bath.
6. Asking them to go to bed.
7. Asking them to do anything that wasn't their idea.
8. Telling them anything you've learned during your multiple years on the planet. They know it already. And more.
9. LOOKING DIRECTLY AT AN INFURIATED TODDLER. Staring at an eclipse of the sun is safer.

TALKING TO ANGRY TODDLERS

Trying to communicate with angry toddlers is kind of pointless. For all of the reasons above. Firstly, looking at them, in order to even talk to them, can go one of two ways: the not-so-good way and the totally disastrous way. Remember, hell hath no fury like a toddler. If you've lost them to Toddler Rage, I suggest, a) walking away; b) walking even further away; c) pretending they aren't yours. Seriously, though, giving them space (as long as they're safe) really does work. I've tried reasoning. Offering them a cuddle. Or a lollipop. When the rage takes hold, they can't see anything but how inept YOU are and they just need a moment to let it all out and then calm down. In a matter of minutes your remorseful (and exhausted) toddler will be accepting your advances and throwing their arms around you, whilst wiping their snot on your shoulder. Most of it comes down to the fact that communication for toddlers is frustrating. They can't talk properly yet and you can't read minds. It's a truly awful combination. Thankfully it doesn't last forever, even though, at the time, it might seem like it does. You can help your toddler feel understood by naming the emotion they're experiencing – sad, cross, scared – and talking to them simply about how this makes them feel. Good luck.

KEEPING YOUR COOL (OR NOT)

You are a human being. With only so much patience. Being tested by an irrational toddler is HARD. Especially when you're tired and under pressure in other ways, which most of us are. If you lose your temper with one (I mean your own, not someone else's), DO NOT BEAT YOURSELF UP. I have done both many, many times and I can assure you there is no salvation or comfort to be found in regret. Move on, kiss and make up and throw yourself into helping them put a jigsaw together back to front, before they lose the plot again and throw all the pieces in different directions (how toddlers do that so spectacularly?). At this point, you've totally done your bit and it is now permissible to lock yourself in the bathroom and eat cake. Ok?

ON THIS DAY

DATE: _____

Accepting that sometimes it is impossible to please a toddler is a real sanity saver.

MY NOTES
(WHAT I LOVED, FELT, WISHED, NEEDED, STRUGGLED WITH, OVERCAME)

....

....

....

....

....

....

....

....

....

....

TO DO LIST

❏ ....

❏ ....

❏ ....

❏ ....

❏ ....

THINGS TO REMEMBER
(THAT I'LL PROBABLY STILL FORGET)

....

....

....

....

....

STUFF THAT ANNOYS YOU
(THIS LIST IS NOT EXHAUSTIVE)

....

....

....

....

....

FUNNY THINGS YOU DID/SAID
(THANKS FOR MAKING ME LAUGH)

....

....

....

....

....

....

....

....

....

....

....

....

....

....

WHAT I WANT YOU TO KNOW
(YEARS FROM NOW)

....

....

....

....

....

....

....

....

....

....

....

....

....

....

We're never meant to
understand toddlers.
We're there to guide them
and keep them safe.
It isn't always easy.

(But just look how
much they love you.)

ON THIS DAY

DATE: _____

No mum has unlimited patience. Go easy on yourself.

MY NOTES
(WHAT I LOVED, FELT, WISHED, NEEDED, STRUGGLED WITH, OVERCAME)

....

....

....

....

....

....

....

....

....

....

....

TO DO LIST

❑ ....

❑ ....

❑ ....

❑ ....

❑ ....

MAKING MOTHERHOOD FUN

IT'S OK TO ADMIT IT

I'm going to let you in on a little secret. No mum enjoys motherhood ALL of the time. Really. Being a mother is neither the most natural thing to all of us nor the most rewarding thing all of the time. Sometimes it *is* really blooming monotonous. And it *is* perfectly fine to acknowledge this. It does not make you a terrible human being. It makes you a real one, with needs and desires of your own. Needs beyond dressing your child. Feeding them. Entertaining them. Feeding them again. Napping them. Bathing them before dragging your sorry, exhausted self across the finishing line to bedtime. There are days, especially when your children are small, when it is hard to even remember what happened between the hours of 7.00 am and 7.00 pm. Did you play with them? Did you really engage with them? Did you have a moment to enjoy this precious day, which we are so often told to cherish? Sometimes it feels impossible amidst everything else that needs doing just to keep them alive, doesn't it?

ROUTINE CAN BE STIFLING

Kids might be happiest in routines. But I'm not sure us mums always are. Routine is all well and good, and it's my personal experience that most kids respond better to a loose structure of some form, but it can sometimes feel overwhelming when you're the one policing it. It can make motherhood feel monotonous and take away the opportunity for fun. When my first two were younger, having been a very routine-based mum from the off, I reached a point where I suddenly felt like a slave to it. I saw that I wasn't enjoying being a mum all that much. That I wasn't much fun to be around. That I was stressed when I could have been relaxed. That I was, well, bored. I was fed up with always *having* to do something. Always having to be somewhere. Always rushing. My days became about ticking the boxes just to make it through the day. Breakfast, tick. Getting dressed, tick. Swimming, tick. Lunchtime, tick. I was never really in the moment with my kids. And they had no idea of the fun person I once was. Because I had never shown them.

DO IT YOUR WAY

We don't want to give up routine altogether, obviously. Kids need to eat at regular intervals and go to bed (eventually). But, these days, I try to make our days more flexible. More forgiving. Having three kids has naturally enforced this because there are so many variables and it is impossible for me to run the tight ship I once did. So what if my boy is wearing his pirate outfit for the fifth day in a row? Or we've all eaten breakfast at different times and only one of those breakfasts contained actual 'breakfast' food? I let a lot go now, but it's taken me so long to see this for the positive development it actually is, rather than berating myself for being 'lazy'. Because it can be really liberating if we accept that, whilst the kids are young at least, there is little time (or need) for us to do this family life *perfectly* and to a rigid timescale. Things will get forgotten amidst the merry chaos. The bins won't get put out. The cats will miss their vaccinations. We may never be domestic goddesses – but how about we settle for being happy ones? Alleviating the frustration or boredom that you feel can be as simple as giving up on something you *should* be doing and doing something else *your* way. Something spontaneous and messy. A breakfast of pancakes when you usually serve porridge. A satisfying Sunday roast out with friends and a 'rebellious' later bedtime than usual. A Friday night movie/sleepover tucked up together in your bed with a takeaway pizza. Anything that makes you feel a little reckless and allows your child to see the fun person you *still* are.

FINDING VALIDATION ELSEWHERE

For many of us, motherhood is not enough in its own right. This might be an inevitable realisation or it may be a disappointing one, which throws you off your path. Discovering you are not completely fulfilled by your role as a mother can be unnerving and lead you to believe you must be a bad one. That we should put ourselves last once we become mothers is one of the biggest (and most damaging) myths we live with today. You've been a woman for far longer than you've been a mother. Why would you suddenly expect to put *her* and her needs aside? For the rest of time, I am a better mother when I am personally fulfilled and when I am doing things to sustain myself. When I remember and nurture that woman within. For me, this can be as simple a task as going for a run or writing. Hitting a goal, no matter how small, can also give me that feeling. You know the one, where your heart soars a little and you feel that sense of satisfaction, contentment and achievement. I've even got it from *finally* putting that pile of washing away that's spent the past few weeks being moved from the kitchen table to the sofa (yes, really). It's all about recognising what makes *you* tick. It's different for each of us but, with practice, you can tap into this at will. There's a whole chapter on this later – 'Small things to lift your mood.' You'll soon be more able to change how you feel in any given moment and create that good energy again.

one thing that makes my heart soar...

....

....

....

....

....

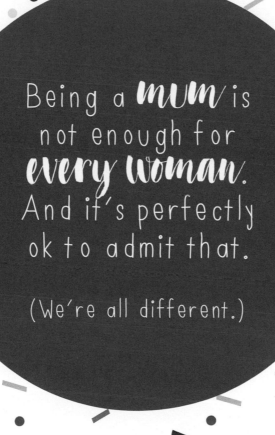

Being a **mum** is
not enough for
every woman.
And it's perfectly
ok to admit that.

(We're all different.)

ON THIS DAY

DATE: _____

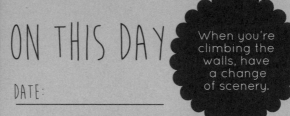

When you're climbing the walls, have a change of scenery.

MY NOTES
(WHAT I LOVED, FELT, WISHED, NEEDED, STRUGGLED WITH, OVERCAME)

....

....

....

....

....

....

....

....

....

....

....

TO DO LIST

❑ ....

❑ ....

❑ ....

❑ ....

❑ ....

THINGS TO REMEMBER
(THAT I'LL PROBABLY STILL FORGET)

....
....
....
....
....

STUFF THAT MAKES ME TICK
(AND MAKES MY HEART SOAR)

....
....
....
....
....

FUNNY THINGS YOU DID/SAID
(THANKS FOR MAKING ME LAUGH)

....
....
....
....
....
....
....
....
....
....
....
....
....

WHAT I WANT YOU TO KNOW
(YEARS FROM NOW)

....
....
....
....
....
....
....
....
....
....
....
....
....

Motherhood loves company. If you're finding things a bit dull and relentless, relieve the boredom and hang out with some other mums in the same boat.

(Jammie Dodgers ~~optional~~ recommended.)

ON THIS DAY

DATE: _____

If you're feeling stifled by routine, have a day off from it and do something FUN.

MY NOTES
(WHAT I LOVED, FELT, WISHED, NEEDED, STRUGGLED WITH, OVERCAME)

....

....

....

....

....

....

....

TO DO LIST

.... ❏ ....

.... ❏ ....

.... ❏ ....

.... ❏ ....

.... ❏ ....

THE SEVEN STAGES OF A TANTRUMING TODDLER

Toddlers know how to tantrum. For the uninitiated (and even the initiated, come to that), a toddler tantrum is mortifying, especially when it happens in public. Here's a tongue-in-cheek guide to help you through. Actually, it won't help you very much at all but it will at least prepare you for what comes next.

STAGE 1: THE STAND-OFF

Position: Child stands defiantly. Won't budge. Stares at you intently.

Scenario: You can almost miss this first stage in the tantruming process. Are they smiling or crying? It's hard to tell. Until they don't move. At all. And perform the stand-off. 'Who's going to give in first. Me or you?' That's what your toddler is thinking right now.

Reason: They're giving you a fair chance to work out what's wrong. To see how good a parent you actually are. This is an IMPOSSIBLE task that you are destined to fail. I mean, it could be anything from the wrong socks to the wrong coat to the wrong type of sunshine. Who the f*** knows?

Solution: Encouraging words (fail). Followed by threats (fail). And, finally, begging with chocolate (you).

STAGE 2: THE WARNING

Position: Much pointing.

Scenario: If the stand-off hasn't worked and you haven't resorted to bribery (well done) your toddler will progress to POINTING. To the thing they want. NOW. But even though they know what they want, you haven't a clue. 'Dat!' they cry. 'Dat!' As you look on dumbfounded.

Reason: Pure frustration that you are such an idiot and are clearly deliberately ignoring what they want.

Solution: Find out what they want and FAST. Before the tantrum progresses to Stage 3.

STAGE 3: THE PRE-MELTDOWN

Position: Toddler rests their head on the floor and sticks their bum in the air (otherwise known as the Tantruming Downward Dog).

Scenario: Things are getting serious. Your toddler is now losing the will to live. They've given you TWO chances to do what they want and you've messed up. TWICE.

Reason: 'WHY ARE YOU DOING THIS TO ME?' (What your toddler would say if they could properly articulate their frustration.)

Solution: Unless you're totally willing to give in to whatever demand your toddler is making (if you've even worked it out), there's pretty much no going back once they've reached this stage. It's now about weathering the storm.

STAGE 4: THE BOUNCE

Position: Bouncing up and down frantically like a demented Tigger.

Scenario: Laying down isn't getting your toddler anywhere. So now they'll try motionnoise. This basically involves jumping up and down in rhythm with their own ever-increasing wails. If you're at home, you're likely thinking about where to hide. If you're out in public, you're probably pretending this child isn't yours.

Reason: Pure rage. At this point your toddler can't even remember what it is they wanted.

Solution: Step away from the toddler. And don't look them in the eye. Whatever you do.

STAGE 5: THE EMOTIONAL APPEAL

Position: Tragically sad face peering up at yours.

Scenario: This is a sure sign your toddler is running out of tactics. So they'll try pulling at your heartstrings. Maybe you'll let them wear their muddy wellies indoors if they show you how much it means to them. Those RSPCA adverts with the sad donkey haven't got anything on your toddler.

Reason: They can't believe you're still in the game. ' have you not caved already?' they're thinking. 'Look how sad I am!'

Solution: Don't fall for it. You've come too far.

STAGE 6: THE HEAD FLIP

Position: A lot of head tossing back and forward, accompanied by possible screaming.

Scenario: They hate you.

Reason: In summary? You've ruined their life. Because you're stubborn and mean and wouldn't let them wear the wellies.

Solution: Adoption.

STAGE 7: THE END

Position: Lying down on the floor, like a dehydrated starfish.

Scenario: Your toddler's exhausted themselves from riding that emotional rollercoaster. There's nothing left to do now but for them to have a little lie down. And sob. Loudly.

Reason: Stages 1–6.

Solution: Step over them. Or wait. Or join them on the floor for a rest. With any luck your toddler will fall asleep where they're lying.

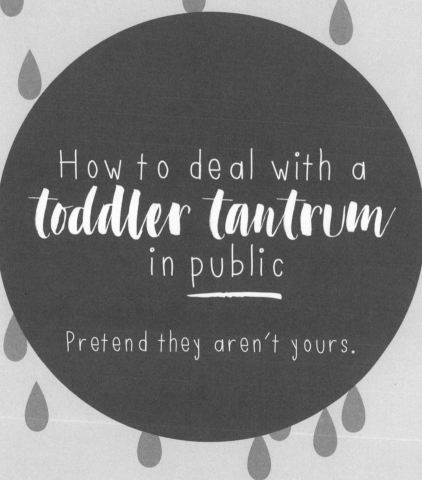

How to deal with a
toddler tantrum
in public

Pretend they aren't yours.

ON THIS DAY

DATE: _____

Could that tantrum actually be hunger, thirst or an overdue nap? (Clutching at straws.)

MY NOTES
(WHAT I LOVED, FELT, WISHED, NEEDED, STRUGGLED WITH, OVERCAME)

....

....

....

....

....

....

....

....

TO DO LIST

❑ ....

❑ ....

....

❑ ....

....

❑ ....

....

❑ ....

....

THINGS TO REMEMBER
(THAT I'LL PROBABLY STILL FORGET)

....
....
....
....
....

TANTRUMS YOU'VE HAD
(AND THE CRAZY REASONS WHY)

....
....
....
....
....

FUNNY THINGS YOU DID/SAID
(THANKS FOR MAKING ME LAUGH)

....
....
....
....
....
....
....
....
....
....
....

WHAT I WANT YOU TO KNOW
(YEARS FROM NOW)

....
....
....
....
....
....
....
....
....
....
....

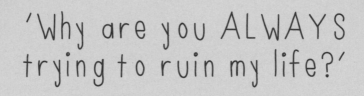

'Why are you ALWAYS
trying to ruin my life?'

(What your toddler thinks
every time you stop them trying
to kill themselves.)

ON THIS DAY

DATE: _____

Never try to rationalise with a toddler. Sometimes not even *they* know what they want.

MY NOTES
(WHAT I LOVED, FELT, WISHED, NEEDED, STRUGGLED WITH, OVERCAME)

....

....

....

....

....

....

....

TO DO LIST

❑ ....

❑ ....

❑ ....

❑ ....

❑ ....

....

....

....

THE 5-7 PM PARENTING SHIFT (THE WITCHING HOURS)

There is a period in *every* day that many (most) parents hate. It starts at about 5.00 pm with dinnertime and ends at around 7.00 pm with bedtime (except it never ends at 7.00 pm. Never.). Some parents call it The Witching Hour (they *wish* it was an hour). Other parents call it, 'How long until I can stop banging my head against the wall?' Here's how it goes.

5.00 PM: DINNERTIME

The hell of dinnertime starts at about 5.00 pm. This is the time when some of us parents are cracking open the wine or eating ALL the sugar; checking Facebook every 1–3 minutes through complete and utter boredom and asking ourselves, 'Do my kids really need to eat dinner *every* day?' We need something (anything) to make the next two hours (Ha ha) remotely bearable. It's like Groundhog Day, but much, much worse because at least Bill Murray only had himself to think about and he got some sleep at night. It's the time when we're most likely to stick pins in our eyes. Because this isn't a Pinterest moment, in which the children eat a variety of coloured foods and jovially chat about their day. It's a moment where they whine and push stuff around their plates, onto the floor and onto each other, whilst we repeat, 'Eat your dinner. Eat your dinner. Eat your dinner,' on loop for 45 minutes like robotic idiots. After which we give up completely and scrape all the leftovers into the bin, take another sip/eat another biscuit and check Facebook again. Just in case anything exciting has happened since we checked it 90 seconds ago. (It hasn't.) Still, the best is yet to come. Bathtime.

6.00 PM: BATHTIME

When you first have a baby (and possibly even before that), you think bathtime will be lovely. Getting your baby all clean, inhaling that delicious baby smell and putting them in a crisp, white baby-gro. You might even use some organic body lotion on them, if you're going all out. Then, a year on – when you're so tired that you can't remember when *you* last had a wash – you give them a sniff and think, 'Do they really need a bath tonight?' before conceding that, yes, they're actually a bit stinky. Or is that you? So in they go! Whilst you sit next to them on the toilet (lid down) and yes, you guessed it, check Facebook. Even though there is nothing to check because you've checked it every 75 seconds since dinnertime. **AND STILL ABSOLUTELY NOTHING NEW HAS HAPPENED**. They flood the bathroom because you're not paying attention. You shout. And that sets the tone for bedtime hour.

6-7.00 PM: THE BEDTIME HOUR

This is the biggest con of ALL time. Because I have never, not once, known The Bedtime Hour to last an hour. Parents don't sit mellow-ly on the sofa with their offspring watching Iggle Piggle float on the sea and Upsy Daisy get in and out of bed. We do alternative stuff like debate what constitutes appropriate nightwear. Pyjamas, yes! Ballerina outfits and fluffy white bear hats, no! And just as we are prepping the kid(s) for the departure to their bedroom with a countdown ('Five minutes to go, now it's three. Ok, you have one more minute.'), the other half comes in from work (or maybe it's you who has missed the first hour and is now sweeping through the door. If so, good call.) 'But I haven't seen them!' says the parent gleefully, in a manner in which only those who haven't spent 12 hours with their kids can muster. They throw them up into the air one by one and there, in that one 'innocent' action, all those futile wind-down efforts are immediately shot to s***. And you're lucky if your child is in bed by 10.00 pm.

ON THIS DAY

DATE: _____

Your child doesn't need a bath EVERY day. (Hurrah!)

MY NOTES
(WHAT I LOVED, FELT, WISHED, NEEDED, STRUGGLED WITH, OVERCAME)

....

....

....

....

....

....

....

TO DO LIST

☐ ....

☐ ....

☐ ....

☐ ....

☐ ....

THINGS TO REMEMBER
(THAT I'LL PROBABLY STILL FORGET)

....

....

....

....

....

BEDTIME BOOKS WE LOVE
(THAT MAKE BEDTIME HAPPIER)

....

....

....

....

....

FUNNY THINGS YOU DID/SAID
(THANKS FOR MAKING ME LAUGH)

....

....

....

....

....

....

....

....

....

....

....

....

....

WHAT I WANT YOU TO KNOW
(YEARS FROM NOW)

....

....

....

....

....

....

....

....

....

....

....

....

....

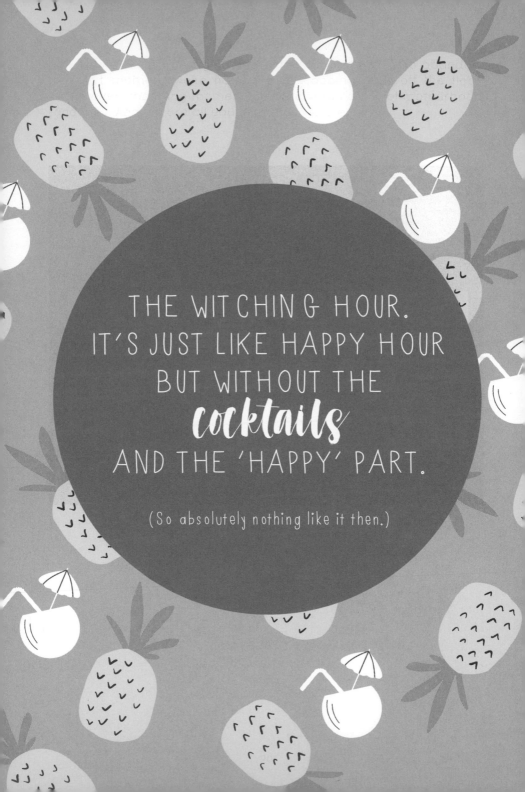

THE WITCHING HOUR.
IT'S JUST LIKE HAPPY HOUR
BUT WITHOUT THE
cocktails
AND THE 'HAPPY' PART.

(So absolutely nothing like it then.)

ON THIS DAY

DATE: _____

You are not alone if you find bedtime is the hardest part of the day NO GUILT.

MY NOTES
(WHAT I LOVED, FELT, WISHED, NEEDED, STRUGGLED WITH, OVERCAME)

....

....

....

....

....

....

....

....

....

....

....

TO DO LIST

❏ ....

❏ ....

❏ ....

❏ ....

❏ ....

NO. YOUR CHILD ISN'T A PSYCHOPATH

IT'S JUST ANOTHER STAGE

At one point or another, we've all wondered, 'Is my child a psychopath?' Ok, maybe not exactly this, although almost every piece of red/black/angry artwork my kids have painted *has* made me ponder whether it's time to call a psychiatrist. When our child behaves anti-socially, it's perfectly natural to a) question whether this is normal; b) panic that your child is going to be a social outcast; and c) doubt everything you've done up until this point. The good news is, it's highly unlikely that, just because your toddler bit/bundled/sat on another child in the playground/nursery, they're going to turn into a psychopath. They're just testing boundaries, and it's another developmental stage you'll fairly soon pass by.

DON'T PANIC

That said, I know that it's still really unpleasant if you have a child that engages in this kind of behaviour. My eldest was one of them. A frequent reoffender from the age of about 18 months right up until she started school. Even now, her default behaviour with her siblings is occasionally physical, when she's frustrated. I fell into all three of the categories above: wondering if she was 'normal' (an irrelevant definition, because what's normal and also, what's so brilliant about being it?); panicking she was going to end up being excluded from things; and comparing myself to other parents who seemed to have such obliging and kind kids. 'Where am I going wrong?' I asked myself often. It made me feel insecure and that I was somehow inadequate as a mother. It definitely caused me to over-parent at times and act upon things that weren't actually that significant because I was so worried she was going to lash out. Several years later, as I watch her grow into a confident, considerate and self-aware young girl, I can now see how many things were just phases and developmental stages. A mere consequence of being so small and testing the waters. In other words, don't panic. It's going to be ok.

ENGAGE POSITIVELY

When your child acts up, it's natural to feel cross with them, especially if another child is involved. In that moment, we're most likely mortified and a bit embarrassed. And we're possibly thinking more of ourselves

> **66** Your child is always your first priority and it's ok to let the rest of the world see that. **99**

than our child, and how their behaviour reflects upon us as mothers. We understandably want to be seen to be doing the right thing, so it's our tendency to jump straight into the situation and discipline our child, whilst fussing over the other one. When we do this, we miss a crucial opportunity to support our child and help them learn. Whether the way in which our child reacted is appropriate, or not, is something we can assess after we've established the reason for their behaviour. Because there's usually one, no matter how small it may seem to us. If we work with our own child first, remove them from the situation and make them feel safe, we've created a calm moment to ask them if they know why they did what they did, before explaining how they could respond differently next time. Toddlers can be told in simple terms things like, 'I can see that was making you sad but we don't hurt others'. Giving your child a chance to explain themselves and allowing them to name (or to hear you name) their frustration or emotion is so important, and it's far more positive than simply assuming your child's in the wrong because we're more focused on what another parent thinks of us. Your child is *always* your first priority and it's ok to let the rest of the world see that.

NEVER COMPARE

One of the most unhelpful things we do as parents is compare our children. Every child is different. We're told this, repeatedly. We know it, deep down. Yet still we fall into the trap of pitting our child against others. Just. Don't. Do. It. It will make you feel miserable and prompt you to react to your child from a negative perspective full of 'lack'. Maybe your child isn't as obedient as you'd like. But how about celebrating that persistent will instead, which earlier saw your toddler finish a puzzle all by themselves? Sometimes it's all in the way we look at it. Choose to reframe a behaviour and see your child's strengths not weaknesses and you'll naturally do this more and more, and praise your child for their positive side. And guess what? They'll do more of that thing rather than the other. It's the old carrot and stick method. There isn't a person in the world who doesn't respond better to encouragement than criticism. On challenging days, when your child's behaviour or your general tiredness makes this feel like a tall order, don't be hard on yourself. If you shout, you shout. If you lose your temper, you lose your temper. If you catastrophise, you catastrophise. It is what it is. Take a breath and put it back into perspective. Reassure yourself, 'We're all different. And we're all exactly as we are meant to be.' Our kids are no exception to this. And there's much peace to be had in realising that. That they are absolutely complete, as they are.

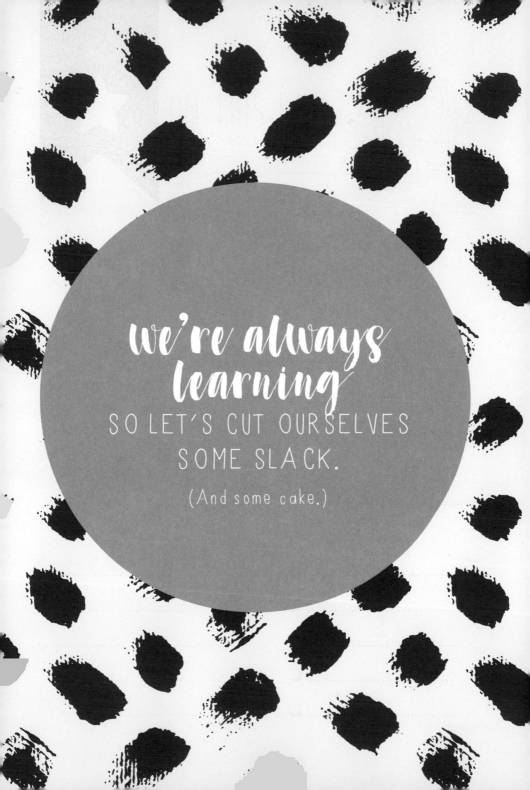

we're always
learning
SO LET'S CUT OURSELVES
SOME SLACK.

(And some cake.)

ON THIS DAY

AMAZING MUM.
AMAZING CHILD.
As you both are.

DATE: _____

MY NOTES
(WHAT I LOVED, FELT, WISHED, NEEDED, STRUGGLED WITH, OVERCAME)

....

....

....

....

....

....

....

....

....

....

....

TO DO LIST

☐ ....

☐ ....

☐ ....

☐ ....

☐ ....

THINGS TO REMEMBER
(THAT I'LL PROBABLY STILL FORGET)

....
....
....
....
....

WHY YOU ARE BRILLIANT
(A LIST OF YOUR STRENGTHS)

....
....
....
....
....

FUNNY THINGS YOU DID/SAID
(THANKS FOR MAKING ME LAUGH)

....
....
....
....
....
....
....
....
....
....
....
....
....

WHAT I WANT YOU TO KNOW
(YEARS FROM NOW)

....
....
....
....
....
....
....
....
....
....
....
....
....

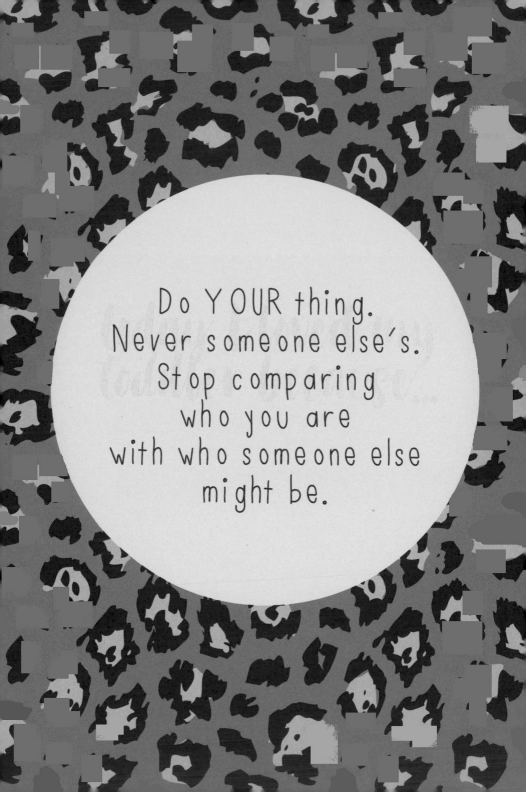

Do YOUR thing.
Never someone else's.
Stop comparing
who you are
with who someone else
might be.

ON THIS DAY

DATE: _____

Focus on your child's strengths to help you through the more challenging times.

MY NOTES
(WHAT I LOVED, FELT, WISHED, NEEDED, STRUGGLED WITH, OVERCAME)

....

....

....

....

....

....

....

....

....

....

TO DO LIST

❑ ....

❑ ....

❑ ....

❑ ....

❑ ....

WHEN YOU FEEL LIKE YOU CAN'T GO ON (YOU CAN)

YOUR HEART WILL GO ON AND ON

I feel the need to quote Celine Dion here (sorry) because there are days when the task of nurturing a small human being feels insurmountable. When you don't know how you're going to get through another long day because you're tired and physically and emotionally spent. And then, just like that, you *do* go on. Because your infinite love for that small human being surpasses everything else (even when they insist on dressing themselves by forcing leggings over their head). It's the greatest love affair you'll ever experience in your lifetime. And it will keep you going through the tough times.

NOTICE THE ORDINARY MOMENTS

Sometimes, when we feel overwhelmed or frustrated, all we need to do is bring ourselves back to the present and notice something joyful. Your child's button nose. Their comedic behaviour. The fact that your child has the luxury of hot water and the sensation of bubble bath on their skin. Parents who suffer the terrible tragedy of losing a child always remark that it's the ordinary moments they miss the most. The slamming of a door. The bickering (yes, really). Putting out a spoon and bowl for breakfast. We all need reminding because motherhood is largely filled with nothing BUT these ordinary moments. Getting kids dressed. Making meals. Doing baths. And we can choose to find some joy in these or we can opt to be bored and frustrated by them. Just saying the words 'ordinary moments' to yourself can be enough of a prompt to ground you and change your focus. Because each and every one of us would live the ordinary moments again and again and again, if it means we get to spend a lifetime with our children.

IT'S OK TO WANT TO ESCAPE

Of course, I still have days where I have no idea how I am going to reach bedtime in one piece. Where I torment myself with fantasies of escaping it all. Going to the airport and hopping on a plane to the Caribbean (I've never even been to the Caribbean). As this is a fantasy that is obviously never going to happen, usually I console myself by eating chocolate digestives behind the kitchen cupboard. It's not comparable, in any way, shape or form, but the (pitiful) rebellion of it sort of helps in that moment. As I've already said (and will keep saying), it's TOTALLY OK to occasionally wish you were doing anything but being someone's mother. It doesn't mean *anything* more than you're struggling temporarily. We all do. So, let it wash over you, don't fight the feeling and enjoy whatever fantasy (or biscuit) it is that takes you away from it all, if only for a moment. Then mix it up a little so you *do* get a realistic chance to escape. Plan a weekend lunch with friends (and no kids), get to that exercise class you've been meaning to try (it will energise you even if you're shattered) or bring their bedtime forward half an hour, have a bath, then get into bed with your Kindle or a good book and 'read-lax'.

IT'S HARDER WHEN THEY'RE YOUNG

One day, when your child is older, more independent and you no longer need to do every little thing for them, you'll look back and be able to see just how intense it actually was looking after someone so small. And what an amazing job you did. This perspective, like so many realisations in motherhood, unfortunately comes too late, when we don't need it quite so desperately. So, to appease any doubts, let me tell you this now. **IT'S INTENSE LOOKING AFTER SOMEONE SO SMALL. YOU ARE DOING AN AMAZING JOB.**

TAKE IT DOWN A NOTCH

When life overwhelms you and you simply don't know where to turn or what to do, that's your prompt to take a step back. From everything you *can* take a step back from. And, when you really start to consider them, it's surprising how many of life's demands and expectations come solely from ourselves. Staying on top of the house. All the admin. Clearing out the toy/clothes cupboards that you've decided *must* be done today. Whatever it is you're currently looking at and thinking, 'I need to sort that', ask yourself this instead, 'Do I *really* need to sort that or, actually, can it wait?' It's so easy to become martyrs in our own lives. We think we need to be the strong one. The capable one. The perfect one. We start to believe that if we want it done right we must do it ourselves. So we bear even more on our small shoulders. It's our bizarre choice to live like this, in motherhood martyrdom. But you know what? We don't have to be everything to everyone. It's impossible and it's unfulfilling. So, hang up your Superwoman pants for a while, do something that lifts your mood and accept you can't do everything. No one can.

KEEP ON SWIMMING

You are capable of marvellous things. But this does not mean you have to be marvellous all of the time. Just keep on swimming downstream because it is tiring and futile to be struggling against the current. Go where the day takes you and accept your feelings, whether good or bad. Because moments pass. If you trust this inevitability you'll also enjoy those similarly fleeting precious moments even more.

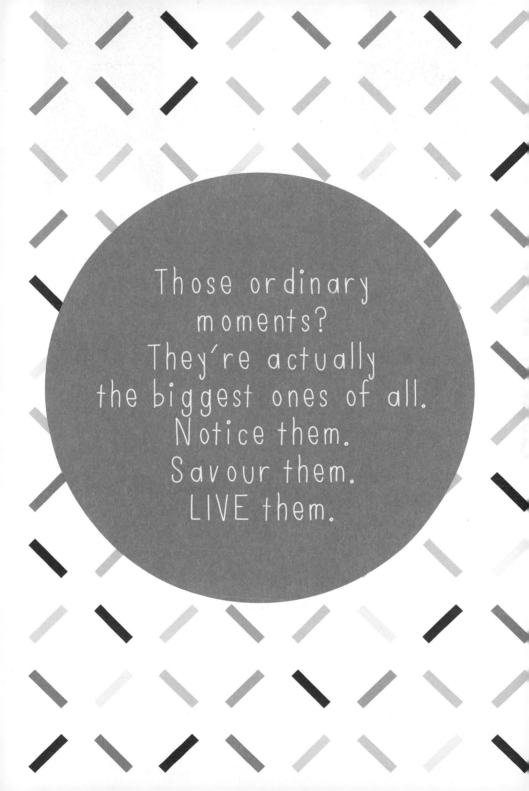

Those ordinary
moments?
They're actually
the biggest ones of all.
Notice them.
Savour them.
LIVE them.

ON THIS DAY

DATE: _____

When you feel that need to escape, do something to lift your mood.

MY NOTES
(WHAT I LOVED, FELT, WISHED, NEEDED, STRUGGLED WITH, OVERCAME)

....

....

....

....

....

....

....

....

....

....

TO DO LIST

☐ ....

☐ ....

☐ ....

☐ ....

☐ ....

THINGS TO REMEMBER
(THAT I'LL PROBABLY STILL FORGET)

....
....
....
....
....

MY PLANS AND FANTASIES
(THINGS I WANT TO DO FOR ME)

....
....
....
....
....

FUNNY THINGS YOU DID/SAID
(THANKS FOR MAKING ME LAUGH)

....
....
....
....
....
....
....
....
....
....
....
....
....
....

WHAT I WANT YOU TO KNOW
(YEARS FROM NOW)

....
....
....
....
....
....
....
....
....
....
....
....
....
....

Sometimes, you wonder how you're going to make it through the day. But no matter how hard it is, it's also as simple as *'I love you, so I will.'*

ON THIS DAY

DATE: _____

The question isn't 'Can you have it all?' But 'Do you really want it all?' SLOW DOWN.

MY NOTES
(WHAT I LOVED, FELT, WISHED, NEEDED, STRUGGLED WITH, OVERCAME)

....

....

....

....

....

....

....

....

....

....

....

TO DO LIST

❑ ....

❑ ....

❑ ....

❑ ....

❑ ....

HOW TO THROW AWESOMELY AVERAGE KIDS' BIRTHDAY PARTIES

SAVE YOUR MONEY (AND YOUR SANITY)

Kids' birthday parties can really suck you in, even from the ripe young age of 2, 3 or 4 years old. Before you even realise what's happened, you've hired a stadium, invited every child (and their sibling) within a 5-mile radius (you didn't want to leave anyone out) and have been frantically trying to reach Ariana Grande's agent to see if she's available for kids' parties. But the truth is that no one needs a party like this. Not least of all a slightly overwhelmed, birthday-shy two-year-old, who will probably spend the entire time clinging to your leg whilst avoiding that slightly scary tissue-paper-donkey-thing hanging from the ceiling. Save your money. There's no need for a Piñata when your guests are so small and light they can barely blow out a candle let alone clobber a papier-mâché mule. In fact, save your money full stop and throw an awesomely average kid's party. THIS is where it's at. It didn't do us any harm, did it?

PARTY LIKE IT'S 1989

Remember when we were growing up? The sorts of parties we had? As a summer baby, my mum just threw us all out in the garden, hoped it didn't rain and did pass the parcel (with just one prize, at the end, not one decadent present per layer). I cried most years. Not because the party was crap, but because it was my party and I could cry if I wanted to. At least at the end of it, as my mum opened a bottle of wine (some things never change in Parent Town), she didn't have to make her peace with the fact she'd spent £5k on the whole shebang. For some reason, kids' parties have taken on a life of their own. They have to be BIG. They have to be BETTER. They have to be at a swanky, innovative venue that no one else has thought of. Bungee-jumping for toddlers, anyone? When your kids are small, my advice is to keep it SIMPLE. Hold off having an actual kid's party, with children, for as long as possible (unless you want to use it as an excuse to see your own pals). Until mine hit three or four, we just had a little tea party at home with family and a couple of close friends. Your child doesn't know any different and you can spend the party budget on some new shoes. Everyone's happy.

HOME IS WHERE THE PARTY IS
Hardly anyone has parties at home anymore. And yet, the few I've been to at someone's house have been more personal than those held in a hall, soft play facility or pizza restaurant. Mainly because when you hire a venue you suddenly decide to invite LOADS of kids, because the hall takes fifty and, well, you may as well make the most of *that*, right? Erm, no. Hosting that many kids in a hall with bad acoustics and fluorescent lighting is enough to induce panic attacks in most adults. When you have the party at home, you have to keep numbers to a minimum: ten kids max. You can use the money you saved on a venue to get an entertainer or, if you're really up for it, do the entertaining yourself with some traditional party games and a craft activity (NO glitter). Pitfalls to watch for are, a) children who want their bottoms wiping whilst you're trying to judge musical statues; b) undercooked chicken nuggets (they don't take a casual 15–18 minutes to cook when you're grilling 100 of the buggers); c) YouTube videos – which you desperately put on whilst cheering on the chicken nuggets – turning wildly inappropriate (Justin Bieber romping about with some girl in a seedy motel room probably isn't the way most parents envisaged tackling the birds and bees talk).

DON'T SUCCUMB TO PEER PRESSURE
So what if your child's friend had a party with actual, real tigers and organic sushi? You had Party Rings AND Hula Hoops and your manky cat poked its head around the door. Don't get into the party comparison stakes. It's amazing how easily you can get drawn in. Remember: awesomely average is the way to go!

ON THIS DAY

Don't let the party pressure get to you. **KEEP IT SIMPLE.**

DATE: _____

MY NOTES
(WHAT I LOVED, FELT, WISHED, NEEDED, STRUGGLED WITH, OVERCAME)

....

....

....

....

....

....

....

....

....

....

....

TO DO LIST

❏ ....

❏ ....

❏ ....

❏ ....

❏ ....

THINGS TO REMEMBER
(THAT I'LL PROBABLY STILL FORGET)

....
....
....
....
....

EASY PARTY IDEAS
(THEMES, GAMES, RECIPES)

....
....
....
....
....

FUNNY THINGS YOU DID/SAID
(THANKS FOR MAKING ME LAUGH)

....
....
....
....
....
....
....
....
....
....
....
....

WHAT I WANT YOU TO KNOW
(YEARS FROM NOW)

....
....
....
....
....
....
....
....
....
....
....

'FORGET
PASS THE PARCEL.
JUST PASS ME
THE WINE.'

(How parents feel after
hosting a kid's party.)

ON THIS DAY

DATE: _____

No mum really enjoys throwing a kid's party. So no guilt if you're relieved when it's over.

MY NOTES
(WHAT I LOVED, FELT, WISHED, NEEDED, STRUGGLED WITH, OVERCAME)

....

....

....

....

....

....

....

....

TO DO LIST

❑ ....

....

❑ ....

....

❑ ....

....

❑ ....

....

❑ ....

AN EASY PEASY BIRTHDAY CAKE WITH WOW FACTOR

I've made a few birthday cakes in my parenting life and this one, probably one of the easiest I've done, completely stole the show. Shame I didn't discover it before the time I spent several hours trying to recreate E.T's bony, glowing finger (I used a slightly massacred red Haribo teddy for the glow, in case you're at all interested).

FOR THE CHOCOLATE SPONGE

4 eggs, beaten
250g butter, softened and cubed
250g caster sugar
175g self-raising flour
75g cocoa powder

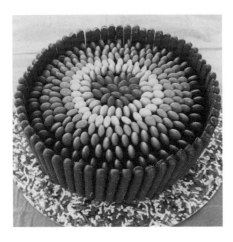

METHOD

1. Set the oven to 180C/Gas Mark 4.

2. Put all the sponge ingredients in a food processor and whizz until mixed. If you don't have a processor, mix the butter and sugar together until pale, stir in the eggs and then slowly combine the flour before mixing in the cocoa powder.

3. Divide the mixture into two 8 inch cake tins (or whatever size you've got), lined with greaseproof paper and bake for approx 18–20 minutes.

4. Remove from the oven and cool. (If you've no greaseproof paper to hand, just butter the cake tins, run a palate knife around the edge when they come out of the oven and tip them out onto a wire rack/plate with a big whack. Technical, I know).

FOR THE ICING

200g icing sugar, sieved
100g butter, softened and cubed
50g cocoa powder
6 tablespoons milk
8 squares dark chocolate

FOR THE DECORATION

3 packs chocolate fingers
8 packs of Smarties, sorted into individual colours

METHOD

1. Mix the icing sugar, butter and cocoa together in a processor or by hand and add the milk.

2. Melt the chocolate in a heatproof bowl over a pan of simmering water (the base of which shouldn't touch the water), cool for a couple of minutes then add to the icing mixture.

3. Spread roughly a third of the icing onto one half of the cake and sandwich the other half on top. Place on a cake board and spread the rest of the mixture over the top and edges of the cake so it is completely covered.

4. Decorate immediately.

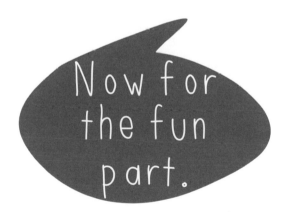

Now for the fun part.

TO FINISH

You'll have already sorted eight packs of Smarties into their individual colours, probably on a rocking Friday or Saturday night, whilst trying not to eat all the chocolate fingers. Ahem. Stick the chocolate fingers into the icing, around the sides of the cake, standing them up like soldiers. Then take the Smarties, stand them on their side edge and stick them in circles, as in the picture. You can change the colour scheme to whatever you like. Keep in a cool place, serve and wait for all the WOWs. Eat any leftover fingers and Smarties (it's your right).

ON THIS DAY

DATE: _____

PARTY TRUTH #1
Kids want sweets.
The End.
(Try organic
apricots
at your own risk.)

MY NOTES
(WHAT I LOVED, FELT, WISHED, NEEDED, STRUGGLED WITH, OVERCAME)

....

....

....

....

....

....

....

....

TO DO LIST

❑ ....

❑ ....

❑ ....

❑ ....

❑ ....

....

....

....

THINGS TO REMEMBER
(THAT I'LL PROBABLY STILL FORGET)

....
....
....
....
....

THANK YOU NOTES
(THAT I'LL HOPEFULLY ACTUALLY SEND)

....
....
....
....
....

FUNNY THINGS YOU DID/SAID
(THANKS FOR MAKING ME LAUGH)

....
....
....
....
....
....
....
....
....
....
....
....

WHAT I WANT YOU TO KNOW
(YEARS FROM NOW)

....
....
....
....
....
....
....
....
....
....
....
....

Take a moment
to remember
the **real** meaning behind
your child's birthday.
That *amazing* day
you brought
them into the world.

ON THIS DAY

DATE: _____

Take a photo of your child opening each present and email it as a 'Thank You'.

MY NOTES
(WHAT I LOVED, FFIT, WISHED, NEEDED, STRUGGLED WITH, OVERCAME)

....

....

....

....

....

....

....

....

TO DO LIST

❏ ....

....

❏ ....

....

❏ ....

....

❏ ....

....

❏ ....

LET'S TALK ABOUT 'WINE O' CLOCK'

MUMS AND BOOZE

Since my parenting journey started nine years ago, somewhere along the way I noticed us mums talking about wine. A LOT. We alternated it with gin, the ultimate Mother's Ruin. And then prosecco. Our Facebook feeds were filled with 'wine o'clock' selfies and comments about the need for that 5.00 pm glass of wine to get us through the bedtime hours. I don't think anyone who ever did (or does) this thought it was 'cool'. I just think it's what we were actually doing. Some of this talk was likely exaggerated or in jest (especially amongst us mummy bloggers – I've made a few flippant remarks myself in this notebook for pure entertainment and relatability). Most of us probably weren't downing a bottle every night, as our social media pages may have implied. But I also know that it is really easy to come to rely on that glass of wine when the days are tough, long and monotonous, and that one glass can very easily turn into two glasses. Three. Or the whole bottle.

THERE'S NOTHING WRONG WITH WINE (UNTIL THERE IS)

I go through periods of drinking and also abstaining. So I am not going to preach that booze is *bad* or *wrong*. I don't believe it is. But I do believe that we need to be aware of our drinking and why we're doing it, and that we have a responsibility to do this for one another. Especially if, like me, you have a tumultuous relationship with alcohol, which could potentially become more sour than sweet. Like many of my generation, in my twenties I was very 'all or nothing', much preferring to binge-drink an unhealthy amount once a week than drink moderately more frequently. So when I became a mum and the social life naturally took a backseat, I compromised with having a glass at home. Having a drink of an evening made me feel like a grown-up. It relieved me from the stresses of the day and marked the point at which I went from 'mum' to 'me' again, which felt very important when my kids were really small and I often questioned my new identity. As I had more kids and they simultaneously reached different stages, each challenging in their own way, I carried on this drinking pattern. I didn't drink every day but, on some days I would drink closer to a bottle. I would find myself thinking about wine or looking forward to it from

4.00 pm onwards, when I started the humdrum routine of dinner-time. I wasn't concerned. Every mum I knew, in real life and virtually, was doing it too. It made it feel very normal and socially acceptable. As mum and author, Clare Pooley, observes in her brilliant book, *The Sober Diaries*, 'you're more likely to be offered a glass of wine at a playdate, than a cup of tea.' Nothing wrong with it at all then, right?

ERM, MAYBE IT'S NOT NORMAL

Then, I hit my personal low point, which still makes me cringe to this very day. I posted a selfie on my 'Surviving Motherhood' Facebook page of me looking fed up, drinking a gin in a can in the park, with my kids playing on the swings behind me. Seeing it in colour, I suddenly became conscious of how wrong that image was, for me, despite hundreds of other mums liking and commenting on it. No one asked WHY I was doing this in a park, instead of playing with my kids: they all 'just got it'. Mums drinking had become the norm. But I felt really uncomfortable about that occasion, and from then on my 'wine' selfies became the exception, not the rule. I realised that we all need to be mindful of the images we're portraying to other mums and the 'normal' motherhood culture we're helping to establish.

SOMETIMES WE DRINK BECAUSE WE'RE BORED

Now that my kids are older and becoming more independent, I can see how much having a teatime drink was, more often than not, rooted in sheer boredom. I did it to numb the experience of serving up another meal that probably no one would eat, before battling bath and bedtime. I'm deliberately painting the bleakest picture and of course not every day was like this, but it never occurred to me at the time that boredom was the reason. That it had just become a habit, which I no longer questioned. I could just as easily have satisfied that boredom with a cup of tea, a chore ticked off the to-do list or 10 minutes on a mindfulness app.

DRINK AND DEPRESSION

Alcohol is a known depressant. So it makes sense that it will aggravate mental health issues such as depression and anxiety, which so many of us suffer from once we become mums. Ironically, drink is the way many of us switch off those anxious thoughts, only for them to come back even louder the next day. I've spoken to many mums who have reduced their drinking or chosen sobriety and every single one has said it has helped their depression and anxiety no end. It's something to bear in mind, if you're predisposed to either.

NEVER ANY JUDGEMENT

It's easy for me to say all of this now. My oldest is nine and my youngest is four. I'm through those intense early years of mother-hood and I did it with the help of booze. So, if you're pouring a glass right now, you feel happy about it and you have it under control, ENJOY THAT TIPPLE. If, on the other hand, you've started to feel a pang of guilt as you open a bottle or it just doesn't make you feel good anymore, acknowledge that there *are* other things you can do to alleviate any boredom or reward yourself. These days, as we're encouraged to embrace the new self-care culture, I'm more likely to be found having a ginger and lemongrass cordial topped with sparkling water followed by a bath and early night with my Kindle. I've seen many of my mum peers doing the same. And I think that's pretty cool.

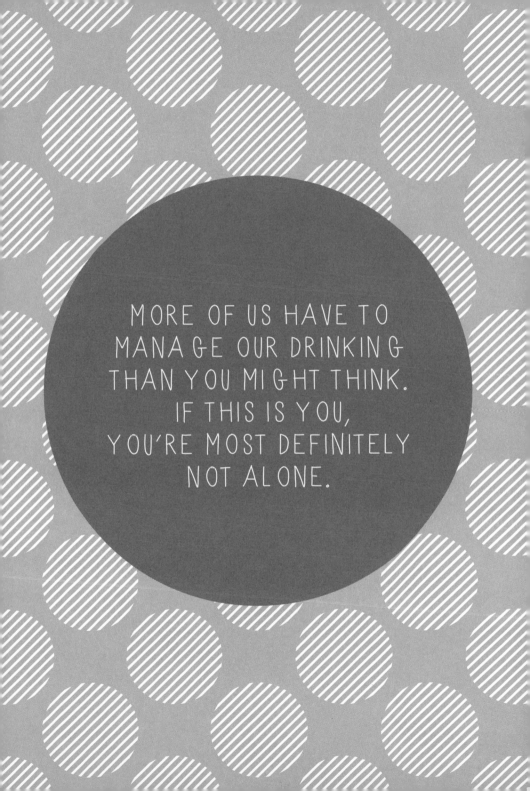

MORE OF US HAVE TO
MANAGE OUR DRINKING
THAN YOU MIGHT THINK.
IF THIS IS YOU,
YOU'RE MOST DEFINITELY
NOT ALONE.

ON THIS DAY

DATE: _____

If something you're doing no longer feels right, change it.

MY NOTES
(WHAT I LOVED, FELT, WISHED, NEEDED, STRUGGLED WITH, OVERCAME)

....

....

....

....

....

....

....

....

....

....

....

TO DO LIST

❑ ....

❑ ....

❑ ....

❑ ....

❑ ....

THINGS TO REMEMBER
(THAT I'LL PROBABLY STILL FORGET)

....
....
....
....
....

STUFF I CAN DO
(TO REWARD OR DISTRACT MYSELF)

....
....
....
....
....

FUNNY THINGS YOU DID/SAID
(THANKS FOR MAKING ME LAUGH)

....
....
....
....
....
....
....
....
....
....
....
....
....
....

WHAT I WANT YOU TO KNOW
(YEARS FROM NOW)

....
....
....
....
....
....
....
....
....
....
....
....
....
....

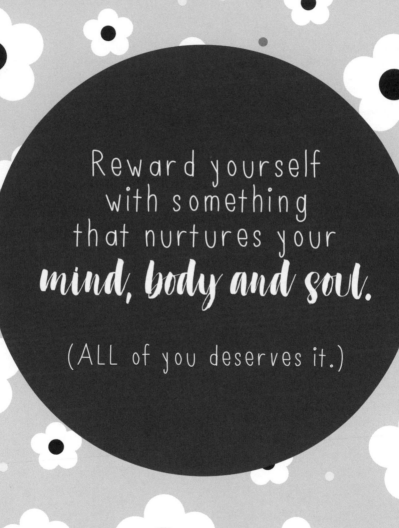

Reward yourself
with something
that nurtures your
mind, body and soul.

(ALL of you deserves it.)

ON THIS DAY

DATE: _____

Want an alternative to that glass of wine? Top up your favourite cordial with sparkling water and a slice of lime.

MY NOTES
(WHAT I LOVED, FELT, WISHED, NEEDED, STRUGGLED WITH, OVERCAME)

....

....

....

....

....

....

....

....

....

....

....

TO DO LIST

❑ ....

❑ ....

❑ ....

❑ ....

❑ ....

GETTING OUT OF THE HOUSE (AND BACK IN AGAIN)

WHY ARE SHOES SUCH A CONUNDRUM?

There are many activities that are *really* fun to do with your kids. One of our most enjoyable is that old favourite – Getting Out of the House (and then back home again). This seems to be a game that doesn't change, no matter how old they are. The aim is to get out of the house in less than 2 hours. I spend at least 45 minutes of this asking the kids to put their shoes on. If I whispered, 'Put your shoes on because we're going to the shops to buy a kilo of sweets,' my kids would not only hear me from two floors up but they'd also miraculously know what a pair of shoes were and where to put them on their bodies. Ask them to do this at ANY OTHER TIME, especially to go to nursery or school, and the utter confusion in their expressions indicates that apparently I am asking FOR THE WORLD. I don't know why it's such a difficult proposition. All I do know is that, once you have children, you'll pretty much ask yourself this daily.

KEEP IT REAL (SIMPLE, AND CHEAP)

In my experience, having fun with kids is about keeping it simple. And cheap – preferably free. As any jaded parent will tell you, it's about setting realistic expectations. For you *and* your child. By realistic, I actually mean LOW. Really, really low. There are many things my kids *still* do not know about, years into their (somewhat underwhelming) childhood. Legoland. Posh Harrods' Santa. That batteries can be replaced. Peer pressure from other parents can make you feel you have to do every age-appropriate activity out there. But the truth is, for my kids at least, that they have always been happiest in our beautiful local park. On their scooters or bikes. Riding up and down hills at vast speeds, like the kids from E.T. (minus the alien). I'm not sure this would be *such* an exciting proposition if I continually overindulged them. Kids don't know how much something cost or whether it's THE thing to be doing right now, especially when they're small. You'll spend the best part of £100+ getting into somewhere like Peppa Pig World and they'll spend the whole time examining a twig. When you *do* decide to splash out and treat them, make sure the activity suits them and their interests. There's no point going to meet the whole cast of *In the Night Garden* if they have a fear of anything dressed up. You're going to spend the whole time with them hiding behind you in terror. Trust me, I've been there.

IT'S ABOUT THE JOURNEY (NOT THE DESTINATION)

Whatever you do when you're out and about with small children, the chances are it won't be perfect. Ditch that delusion, once and for all. Be patient. Allow plenty of time to cover the shortest distance (and yes, it *is* excruciating). Even now, our excursions are often fraught with drama. On the way to the park, someone will lose a hairband (DISASTER) or graze a knee and we will spend 20 minutes retracing the paltry forty steps we've managed to take or administering a bandage. There have been occasions when, by the time we've reached the park, it's almost been nightfall, and after 5 minutes on the swings it's time to go. Ninety minutes and sixty-three tantrums later, we actually manage to leave the park and start the long, arduous journey home. With only one shoe. What was it that a 'wise' person once said? 'It's about the journey, not the destination.' Mmmm. I bet they never did the journey with a volatile two- or three-year-old.

BRILLIANT THINGS TO DO WITH YOUR KIDS

You can't beat venturing into The Great Outdoors with kids. With three of them in tow, I always favour open spaces, where I can relax a little bit and not have to keep track of them amidst a million other people. Parks (there are so many to visit, mix it up!). Woodlands (great for exploring and collecting stuff). One of the amazing Gruffalo Trails (find your local one online). A trip to the seaside with ice creams and good old-fashioned fish and chips on the beach at the end of a sunny, salty day (just watch out for giant seagulls swiping your bewildered child's cheese roll straight from their hand). Give them a list of natural things to find and then go home and collage them (I'm a truly rubbish 'craft mum' and even I have managed this). Easy days like this are what the best memories are made of.

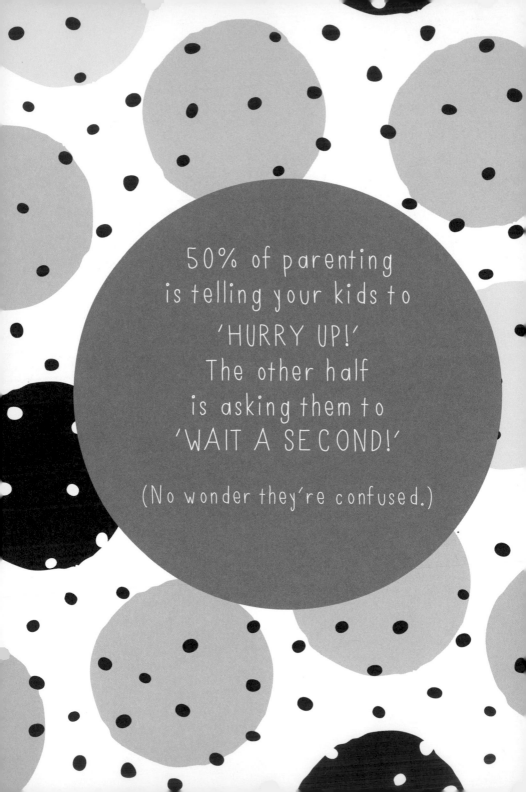

50% of parenting
is telling your kids to
'HURRY UP!'
The other half
is asking them to
'WAIT A SECOND!'

(No wonder they're confused.)

ON THIS DAY

DATE: _____

Your child never needs impressing. Your company is all they want.

MY NOTES
(WHAT I LOVED, FELT, WISHED, NEEDED, STRUGGLED WITH, OVERCAME)

....

....

....

....

....

....

....

TO DO LIST

....

□ ....

....

□ ....

....

□ ....

....

□ ....

....

□ ....

ON THIS DAY

DATE: _____

Days out together are precious time for you and your child, without any distractions.

MY NOTES
(WHAT I LOVED, FELT, WISHED, NEEDED, STRUGGLED WITH, OVERCAME)

....

....

....

....

....

....

....

....

TO DO LIST

❏ ....

❏ ....

❏ ....

❏ ....

❏ ....

....

....

....

THINGS TO REMEMBER
(THAT I'LL PROBABLY STILL FORGET)

....
....
....
....
....

BRILLIANT PLACES TO GO
(THAT WE CAN ENJOY TOGETHER)

....
....
....
....
....

FUNNY THINGS YOU DID/SAID
(THANKS FOR MAKING ME LAUGH)

....
....
....
....
....
....
....
....
....
....
....
....

WHAT I WANT YOU TO KNOW
(YEARS FROM NOW)

....
....
....
....
....
....
....
....
....
....
....
....

today

is tomorrow's memory.

(Make the most of the time
before they start school.)

ON THIS DAY

DATE: _____

Take life at your child's pace for a while. You'll feel less frustrated.

MY NOTES
(WHAT I LOVED, FELT, WISHED, NEEDED, STRUGGLED WITH, OVERCAME)

....

....

....

....

....

....

....

....

....

....

....

TO DO LIST

❑ ....

❑ ....

❑ ....

❑ ....

❑ ....

10 INDOOR ACTIVITIES TO KEEP THEM (AND YOU) HAPPY

You can't *always* get out and about. When bad weather stops play. Or illness. Or general fatigue means you just can't face playing Getting Out of the House again that week. On days like this, CBeebies or Netflix will only go so far and eventually you'll need to amuse them, somehow. Here are some easy suggestions that any mum can do even if, like me, you're totally allergic to pipe cleaners.

1. Make milkshakes. Let your child pick some ingredients and blend it up. Then pretend to drink yours. Mmmmmm.

2. Make (and eat) pancakes for breakfast. We do this a lot in our house. The kids help. Then I let them go wild and decorate them with whatever we have in the kitchen. Chocolate sauce. Strawberry sauce. Honey. Sprinkles. Raisins. Bananas. Seeds. I'll be honest, the pancakes look pretty vile by the time they've finished with them. And it takes me about 3 hours to 'unsticky' all the surfaces and all the errant flour that's made its way into every crevice. But it makes them SO happy.

3. Have a car disco. This sounds bonkers. Because it is. But it's perfect for a rainy day. Basically, you sit in the car, turn the radio up and everyone dances around like loons. My kids think it's hilarious. And I would be lying if I said I didn't get a kick out of it too.

4. Make slime. My kids would do this all day long. And it's super easy. PVA glue (three big squeezes), shaving foam (couple of squirts) and a teaspoon of Optrex eye solution. Simply pour the glue into a pot, add the shaving foam and the Optrex and mix until you can knead it without it sticking to your fingers. It's a bit of trial and error to get the right consistency. You can add food colouring, paint or even glitter to really bling it up (coming out in hives yet?).

5. Melting chocolate. Simply melt 100g of dark or milk chocolate, 30g of butter and 100g of honey/golden syrup in a bowl set over a simmering pan of water (the base of which isn't touching the water). Allow to cool slightly then add whatever you like – crushed biscuits, raisins or other dried fruit, mini marshmallows . . . there are no limits here. You can either eat it 'raw' with a spoon or put it into a cake tin, lined with cling film and refrigerate for a couple of hours. You'll then have your very own impromptu Rocky Road. Which you can eat, when your child isn't looking.

6. Memory games. For them, not you. Although, if your memory's anything like mine, this might benefit you too. I personally find board games with kids under four quite challenging. We've played Guess Who? several times, only to find out at the end that Claire, despite wearing a hat AND glasses (basically the jackpot in Guess Who?, right?), may as well be a bald old man, according to my youngest. Those memory games with the boards and little cards, however, are really easy to understand. Help your child fill their trolley with all of the items on their shopping list. (Or watch them lose complete concentration and throw all the pieces around the room.)

7. Role play. You can't beat a game of doctors and nurses. You get to be the patient. And to lay down whilst your child hits you over the head with various objects and pokes things into your mouth. It's ok, though, because they'll warn you first, 'This is going to hurt.' You can enjoy all the 'pampering', whilst you ponder how the NHS will be lucky, lucky, lucky if your child decides to pursue a career in nursing.

8. Paint. Ok, it's a bit messy and you'd far rather the nursery/child-minder/grandparents do it. BUT. My kids practically foam at the mouth when I get the paints out. And they'll sit there for ages, until the yellow has gone a dark shade of brown. My top tip: DO NOT leave children unsupervised in this activity, no matter how old they are, unless you want some artistic input on your walls/floor or are happy to see their younger brother/sister turned into a (slightly brown) Minion or (very blue) Smurf.

9. Enjoy a lazy morning. There are NO prizes for getting out of the house early. We know this. So, ditch the mum guilt. Grab some cushions and a duvet and make a giant bed in the lounge – or just all crowd into your actual bed with some books. You'll probably get bounced on but it's a great way to have some safe rough and tumble time with your small person.

10. Ask your child what THEY want to do and then do it. This one is risky. You could end up being Captain Hook for the rest of time. Playing with your kids doesn't come naturally to a lot of us. I'm sure this is why we throw money at baby sensory classes and the like. If the thought of playing with your child brings on The Fear, you are not alone. When I asked a group of mums what they felt most guilty about, not playing with them enough topped the list. Also, not wanting to play with them enough. And not losing themselves in the activity when they did play, whilst secretly counting down the minutes until they could do something else. DO NOT FEEL BAD ABOUT THIS, if this is you. We aren't two-, three- or four-year-olds. Playing isn't as instinctive to us as it is to them. Every now and then, though, stop what you're doing and give them as little as 5 minutes of your time. It will mean the world to them. And it will lift your mood, too.

So there you have it; 10 indoor activities to keep you both happy. And I didn't so much as mention a pipe cleaner.

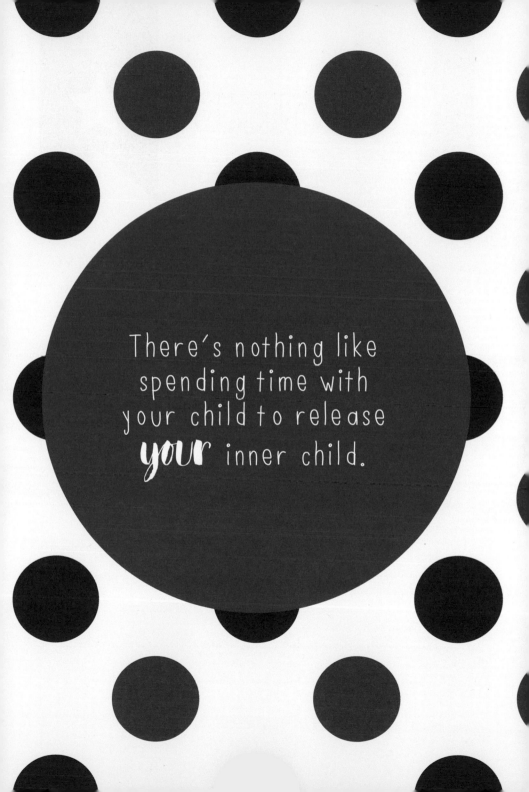

There's nothing like spending time with your child to release *your* inner child.

ON THIS DAY

DATE: _____

If you find playing boring, don't feel bad. Lots of mums do.

MY NOTES
(WHAT I LOVED, FELT, WISHED, NEEDED, STRUGGLED WITH, OVERCAME)

....

....

....

....

....

....

....

....

....

....

....

TO DO LIST

☐ ....

☐ ....

☐ ....

☐ ....

☐ ....

THINGS TO REMEMBER
(THAT I'LL PROBABLY STILL FORGET)

....
....
....
....
....

BRILLIANT THINGS TO DO
(WHEN WE WANT/NEED TO STAY IN)

....
....
....
....
....

FUNNY THINGS YOU DID/SAID
(THANKS FOR MAKING ME LAUGH)

....
....
....
....
....
....
....
....
....
....
....
....
....

WHAT I WANT YOU TO KNOW
(YEARS FROM NOW)

....
....
....
....
....
....
....
....
....
....
....
....

Kids really just want
to be with us.
So *involve* them in
whatever you're doing.
Washing. Tidying. Cooking.

(Just be together.)

ON THIS DAY

DATE: _____

Every now and again say 'Yes' instead of 'Wait a minute'.

MY NOTES
(WHAT I LOVED, FELT, WISHED, NEEDED, STRUGGLED WITH, OVERCAME)

....

....

....

....

....

....

....

....

....

....

....

TO DO LIST

☐ ....

☐ ....

☐ ....

☐ ....

☐ ....

WHY DO WEEKENDS (SOMETIMES) SUCK?

A LOVELY FAMILY WEEKEND?

Weekends as a family can be lovely. Or, sometimes, they can be really hit or miss. I'm going to address the latter here (the worst scenario) because, let me assure you, EVERYONE feels like this at some point or other (even if they pretend otherwise). In the early years, weekends can take some getting used to and require some low-key organisation and communication for everyone to be happy. When you've spent all week desperately looking forward to a couple of days all together, whether you've been home alone with a small person or at work without them, it can be really disheartening when Saturday morning arrives and you get off on the wrong foot. You can't work out why it isn't more straightforward than this. Weekends are supposed to be *fun*, right? This is what you dreamed of when you threw away the condoms, got all gooey eyed and said to each other, 'Let's have a baby.' A lovely, family weekend. So why do they sometimes suck?

WEEKENDS WITH KIDS ARE DIFFERENT

Before kids, you may have had a leisurely weekend breakfast at 11.00 am. Perhaps a brunch out – with a slight hangover. Fast forward to life after kids and the reality is three separate sittings of soggy Weetabix, Rice Krispies without milk (you've run out) and burnt toast at 6.30am. Plus a few tantrums because the Rice Krispies aren't Coco Pops. You will have substituted shopping/sport/laying on the sofa hungover for a day at an overpriced farm with subdued llamas. 'Happy Hour' has been replaced by 'Bedtime Hour' – as we've established, it is neither happy nor an hour and you are considering suing under the Trade Descriptions Act. This isn't quite what you had in mind. Well, weekends with kids *are* different. The End. Best to make your peace with this immediately (if you haven't already), enjoy them for what they are and try to go with the flow. Because, actually, hanging out with that small person you made together is pretty cool. And weren't those hangovers just *really* horrendous? Who misses them?

IT'S MORE NORMAL THAN YOU MIGHT THINK

You're not alone if, by 9.00 am, you want to decapitate your other half or just have a good old moan at them. All around the country, the same scenario is playing itself out. Again and again. Like so much, it comes down to expectations and, very often, mismatched ones. The parent who has worked all week might be tired and looking forward to an actual, leisurely weekend, remembering the weekends of days gone by and possibly momentarily forgetting the pint-sized toddler who's going to make for a very different reality. It can take time to reacclimatise to the world of parenting, when you've been largely out of it all week. Meanwhile, the parent who has been at home with said pint-sized toddler is probably desperate for a break and looking to their partner to provide this (before getting frustrated when their partner doesn't seem to realise this. At all). If you've *both* been out working then you might *both* be feeling a bit out of your depth, alongside a toddler who's equally tired from a busy week in childcare. In summary: whatever your home/work/parenting dynamic, weekends take a bit of adjustment every single week – to understand one another, to all be around one another, to get back in the groove again. When we allow ourselves to do this, when we stop wishing for what simply isn't and accept what is, the way we approach the weekend changes dramatically and for the better.

PARENTING TOGETHER CAN BE CONFUSING

Another source of weekend conflict is how you parent together. You might naturally do this well. Or you might be really dire at it, because you don't do things in the same way. Few of us do. Everything your other half does has the potential to irritate you, especially if you're the primary care-giver who usually holds the fort during the week. It can cause serious friction between couples. Why are they doing it like that? Why aren't they listening to what you're *telling them* to do? But the fact is that everyone likes to do things their own way and there isn't a right way to make pasta and cheese. So, let your partner have free rein with your child. Let them work stuff out for themselves and take a back seat for a while. Enjoy the break! If it's just too painful for you to watch and you can't bite your tongue, go and have a shower in peace, or nip out for a coffee. But it's really important that you both have a proper stake in this parenting lark and that you help facilitate this by stepping back. This way, your partner doesn't feel like a spare part or that everything they do is wrong in your eyes.

PUT DOWN YOUR PHONES

One of the biggest bug-bears between couples is the constant use of mobiles, with one partner getting cross because the other is 'chilling out', sitting on the sofa looking at Facebook or Instagram whilst the other is doing everything else. It's an innocent habit, without malice, but it has the potential to promote a (damaging) lack of respect and consideration. And, as we all know, our phones suck up precious time quicker than an errant Dyson, so whilst you think you've only been on there for 10 minutes, it's actually been an hour. Even when you're not using it, a phone's presence – the temptation to scroll: arghhh! – is a continual interruption. There's only one solution to this. PUT DOWN YOUR PHONES and get on with the day ahead of you without them. You don't realise how distracted and disengaged you actually are with your real life until you do this and focus on what's in front of you: your lovely little family.

TALK TO ONE ANOTHER

Finally, there's one simple way for you both to get what you desire. Tell each other. Mismatched expectations come when neither of you have said *out loud* what you'd like out of the weekend or how you see it working. How does your other half know you were hoping they'd take the toddler to the park so you can tidy the house (or have a moment alone and breathe), if you haven't asked them? Likewise, if someone's hoping to catch some sport on the TV later, mentioning this ahead of time means you're both prepared and there are no (angry) surprises later on. It's *all* about considering one another in *everything* you do, because you're raising a child together. Do this and there's room for everyone to feel fulfilled at the end of a busy, family weekend. Communication is key. Otherwise, you'll just end up stomping around passive-aggressively, huffing and puffing. Leave that behaviour to your toddler. They do it way better than you ever can.

SOME FAMILIES SEEM
PERFECT 'WEEKEND FAMILIES'.
IF YOU ARE THE 'OTHER'
KIND, DON'T WORRY. THE FIRST
KIND DON'T REALLY EXIST.

(You just missed witnessing
their meltdown).

ON THIS DAY

DATE: _____

Tell your partner what you'd like from them. Manage one another's expectations.

MY NOTES
(WHAT I LOVED, FELT, WISHED, NEEDED, STRUGGLED WITH, OVERCAME)

....

....

....

....

....

....

....

....

TO DO LIST

....

☐ ....

☐ ....

☐ ....

☐ ....

☐ ....

THINGS TO REMEMBER
(THAT I'LL PROBABLY STILL FORGET)

....
....
....
....
....

MY 'IMPERFECT' WEEKEND
(WHAT I WOULD LIKE IT TO LOOK LIKE)

....
....
....
....
....

FUNNY THINGS YOU DID/SAID
(THANKS FOR MAKING ME LAUGH)

....
....
....
....
....
....
....
....
....
....
....
....
....

WHAT I WANT YOU TO KNOW
(YEARS FROM NOW)

....
....
....
....
....
....
....
....
....
....
....
....

ACCEPT THAT WEEKENDS
ARE WHAT THEY ARE
AND GO WITH THE 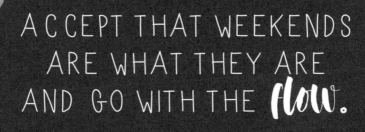.

(You'll stop feeling
disappointed that way.)

ON THIS DAY

Every family is unique. Isn't yours WONDERFUL?

DATE: _____

MY NOTES
(WHAT I LOVED, FELT, WISHED, NEEDED, STRUGGLED WITH, OVERCAME)

....
....
....
....
....
....

....

....

....   **TO DO LIST**

....   ☐ ....

....   ☐ ....

....   ☐ ....

....   ☐ ....

                                              ☐ ....

THE FIVE STAGES OF MOTHERHOOD

STAGE ONE: OPTIMISM

This stage occurs pre-motherhood. Possibly even before you're pregnant. When the thought of a baby is just that – an idyllic thought. You and your partner will both muse on how wonderful it will be to create another being together, with your eyes and their sense of humour. You will want your child to have the best of everything. So you'll buy the latest in buggy technology, even though you need an A level just to work out how to open it. It will sit in the lounge looking all crisp and new and you'll vow to wash the covers regularly and keep the wheels clean. (Ha ha.) The lounge is actually the best place for it because once you drive it off the forecourt, you can kiss goodbye to £950 of the £1,000 you paid for it, as it becomes encrusted in mud, puke and soggy rusks. Not to mention the serious bodywork issues as a result of all the times you'll try to open it one-handed, whilst talking a toddler down from a tantrum, before flinging the damn thing across the car park. In front of an audience. During this 'baby planning' stage you will look permanently wistful and gooey-eyed and say things like, 'Let's try for a baby,' whilst rubbing your non-pregnant stomach. You will look at other people's children with disdain before remarking that 'our child will never be like that'. Your fictional, imaginary child might not be. But your real one? It will probably be worse.

STAGE TWO: SHOCK

This stage happens after birth (and may last until your youngest has gone to school). You'll wander around in a bubble feeling as though you have been plucked from your life and shoved into an alternate reality where the only other women you meet are exactly like you, with limited vocabulary and that slightly harrowed, vacant look of the sleep-deprived. The lights are on, but there's no one home.

STAGE THREE: MOOD SWINGS

This stage goes hand in hand with stage two, because once you get used to the shock factor of motherhood ('Yes, you do have to do this all again tomorrow'), it is common to want to cry at the sheer overwhelmingness of it all whilst simultaneously worrying that you will die and leave your kids with your partner who can't even do a pony tail. These thoughts will keep you awake at 3.00 am (if you ever got to sleep in the first place), meaning you are constantly knackered and particularly susceptible to MOOD SWINGS. These are fun for everyone, particularly your other half, who watches in bewilderment as you rant, cry, scream and laugh in the space of 60 seconds. They call it 'crazy', you call it 'emotional multi-task-ing'. There will be days when you wonder who you are and forget who you used to be. Don't worry, THIS IS PERFECTLY NORMAL and nature's way of not rubbing salt in the wound. I mean, who wants to be reminded that they once had lots of freedom and very little responsibility? You'll totally learn how to manage this with the help of other lovely mums who are every bit as forgetful as you. Which leads me to the next stage – and possibly the most important.

STAGE FOUR: MUM FRIENDS

THANK GOODNESS FOR MUM FRIENDS. Because who else gets it like another mum? The craziness? The desire to sometimes run for the hills whilst loving your kids so much you think you might die anyway? Mum friends never judge. They have your back. They make you feel normal about all the bonkers stuff you're feeling. Because they're feeling it too.

STAGE FIVE: LOVE

This stage is the biggest contradiction of them all. Because whilst you are feeling all the other many emotions, there is another, more overpowering one simmering away in the background that never goes away. LOVE. Yes, you will love your kids SO BLOODY MUCH that if someone offered you a million pounds for each of them you'd probably only sell one. Because although they've completely altered your mind, your body and your life, they've also completely made it. And you couldn't imagine being without them. (Even though you spend at least 5 minutes of every day doing just that.)

ON THIS DAY

DATE: _____

Motherhood. We are ALWAYS learning.

MY NOTES
(WHAT I LOVED, FELT, WISHED, NEEDED, STRUGGLED WITH, OVERCAME)

....

....

....

....

....

....

....

....

TO DO LIST

❏ ....

❏ ....

❏ ....

❏ ....

❏ ....

THINGS TO REMEMBER
(THAT I'LL PROBABLY STILL FORGET)

....
....
....
....
....

WHY I LOVE BEING A MUM
(FOR WHEN I NEED TO REMEMBER)

....
....
....
....
....

FUNNY THINGS YOU DID/SAID
(THANKS FOR MAKING ME LAUGH)

....
....
....
....
....
....
....
....
....
....
....
....

WHAT I WANT YOU TO KNOW
(YEARS FROM NOW)

....
....
....
....
....
....
....
....
....
....
....

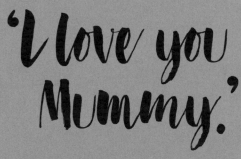

'I love you Mummy.'

(And just like that, it's all worthwhile.
Even the bits that, erm, aren't.)

ON THIS DAY

DATE: _____

On crazy days where you feel you're losing your mind, remember: you are still YOU.

MY NOTES
(WHAT I LOVED, FELT, WISHED, NEEDED, STRUGGLED WITH, OVERCAME)

....

....

....

....

....

....

....

....

TO DO LIST

- ☐ ....

....

- ☐ ....

....

- ☐ ....

....

- ☐ ....

....

- ☐ ....

THE NOT-SO-NEW MUM'S 'NO-SUGAR NO-COOK' GRANOLA BAR

When you don't want to reach for the sugar or you want to nurture your body and soul, these are an amazing (and very satisfying) alternative. They take just minutes to prepare and will totally kick that sugar craving to the kerb. Your child will love them too (and not just because they're on your plate).

INGREDIENTS

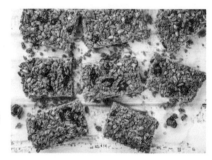

75g porridge oats
4 tablespoons maple syrup/honey
2 tablespoons peanut butter
(crunchy is best)
75g dried fruit
(I used raisins and cut-up apricots)
Smidgen of butter

METHOD

1. Heat the oven to 180°C/Gas Mark 4 and toast the oats on a baking tray for 10 minutes. You can actually bypass this step if you don't mind them not being so crunchy.

2. Melt the syrup and peanut butter together in a pan over a low heat then remove from the heat and mix in the oats and dried fruit.

3. Press into a lightly buttered tin or tupperware (whatever you have to hand!). You can use the bottom of a glass to do this: the mixture should become compacted and firm. Put in the freezer for 20 minutes.

4. Remove. Cut into squares. Tuck in! Store in an airtight container in the fridge.

IT IS NEVER DECADENT
TO INVEST SOME TIME IN

you.

(Think of it as a necessity
not a luxury.)

ON THIS DAY

DATE: _____

Eating well when you can will help your energy levels and give you the strength to POWER ON.

MY NOTES
(WHAT I LOVED, FELT, WISHED, NEEDED, STRUGGLED WITH, OVERCAME)

....

....

....

....

....

....

....

....

....

....

....

TO DO LIST

❏ ....

❏ ....

❏ ....

❏ ....

❏ ....

THINGS TO REMEMBER
(THAT I'LL PROBABLY STILL FORGET)

....
....
....
....
....

HEALTHY SNACK IDEAS
(FOR BOTH OF US)

....
....
....
....
....

FUNNY THINGS YOU DID/SAID
(THANKS FOR MAKING ME LAUGH)

....
....
....
....
....
....
....
....
....
....
....
....
....

WHAT I WANT YOU TO KNOW
(YEARS FROM NOW)

....
....
....
....
....
....
....
....
....
....
....
....

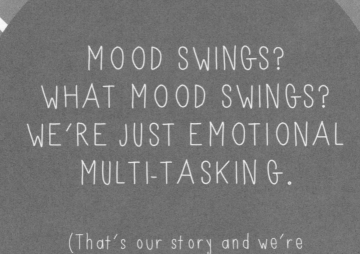

MOOD SWINGS?
WHAT MOOD SWINGS?
WE'RE JUST EMOTIONAL
MULTI-TASKING.

(That's our story and we're
sticking to it.)

ON THIS DAY

DATE: _____

Sugar can aggravate hormones AND anxiety. Lay off it if you're feeling wobbly.

MY NOTES
(WHAT I LOVED, FELT, WISHED, NEEDED, STRUGGLED WITH, OVERCAME)

....

....

....

....

....

....

....

....

....

....

TO DO LIST

❑ ....

❑ ....

❑ ....

❑ ....

❑ ....

THE MUM'S (SLIGHTLY CRAP) GUIDE TO 'ETIQUETTE'

You used to do stuff by the book. Then you had a child, and maybe one or two more, and suddenly you became a bit crap/rude/utterly nuts. Here's how to do the etiquette stuff (without hiring your own PA).

SENDING THANK YOU CARDS

Scenario: Someone very kindly thought about your child. They took the time to pick a gift, wrap it and possibly even post it. Some 4-20 weeks later, you realise you haven't even thanked them. You berate yourself for being so rude, make a note to send them a thank you card. And swiftly forget. Because the toddler has just wet himself. The dog has been sick on the floor. And you've just trodden in it. (Or any scenario a bit like that.) If, by some small miracle, you do get around to writing a thank you card, the chances of you finding a stamp AND actually managing to post it (before someone's scribbled all over it or hidden it) are so slim that you may as well have not bothered in the first place. Next time you see the kind, present-giving person, you'll do the only thing you can and blame 'blooming Royal Mail'. I have sent Christmas thank you cards in May. Yet I'm not sure the phrase 'Better late than never' really applies here.

What you can do instead: Accept you're NEVER going to send an actual thank you card, take a photo of your child with the present at time of opening and text/email it with a little message. Efficient.

ACCEPTING PARTY INVITATIONS

Scenario: Sadly these are not parties you're invited to. You'd be accepting those in a flash. No, these are parties for your child. Which is probably why you're so tardy in responding. You'll eventually reply. When you're chased. Tut. Tut. Tut.

What you can do instead: Check your diary (even though checking your calendar is somehow such a laborious effort) and reply immediately. Done.

DOING STUFF YOU SAID YOU'D DO

Scenario: You absolutely meant to do whatever it was you said you'd do. But it just. Didn't. Happen. Newsflash for all us busy (crap) mums. The only way we'll actually do that stuff is by actually doing it.

What you can do instead: Never say you'll do anything. Then if you *do* do something, it's a lovely surprise for everyone (especially you).

REPLYING TO TEXTS

Scenario: If you don't reply immediately, you're doomed. The text will disappear into the vortex of lonely texts that no one has ever replied to. Leaving you looking rude/insensitive/selfish.

What you can do instead: If you don't have time to reply, don't open them, then at least they'll remain unread and the annoying notification number will prompt you to read it eventually.

JUSTIFYING THE PRESENTATION OF YOURSELF/YOUR KIDS/YOUR HOUSE

Scenario: One of your kids is wearing hot pants. In winter. You, yourself, are wearing slightly (very) stained leggings that you've 'freshened' up with a baby wipe. And your house looks like you've been burgled.

What you can do instead: Never apologise. There's no need to be 'perfect'. This is currently what life looks like on a good day. And that's ok. One day you and the hoover will get friendly again. Or not. People who love you never care about this stuff.

KEEPING TRACK OF NURSERY/WORK/LIFE EVENTS

Scenario: It all starts off well enough. You lay out your child's clothes the night before. And your own, if you're going to work. You put their nursery bag by the door. Fill out any contact books. Remember which day your child has to go as a superhero for Children In Need. Fast forward a couple of years (months) and you sort of lose the plot. There's so much to remember that you always forget something. And it's a bit like breaking your vow not to eat chocolate with just one Malteser and then eating the whole bag in 30 seconds flat. Once you've forgotten one thing, you kind of give up even trying to be efficient.

What you can do instead: Get a whiteboard, stick it on the front of a kitchen cupboard and WRITE EVERYTHING on it. Encourage your partner to get involved in this too, especially if you're both working. You could try sharing tasks. Maybe they do more of the household chores and admin, freeing up your headspace to do the other life/family stuff. Whatever works for you.

BEING EARLY/BEING LATE/NOT TURNING UP AT ALL

Scenario: Your timekeeping is shocking. You either turn up super early because the kids got up at 5.00 am and, 'Well, we thought we'd just get out of the house. Oh sorry, is it only 8.00 am? What time did you want us?' Or you turn up hideously late and barely even realise/remember to apologise. Or, you don't turn up at all. Because... no reason actually. You probably just didn't write it down or look at that flipping calendar.

What you can do instead: Buy a watch. Use that whiteboard! Or never accept an invitation anywhere, that way you'll never be early/late/not turn up at all.

ENTERTAINING ACTUAL PEOPLE

Scenario: You used to be so proper. Ok, that's a bit of an exaggeration. But you used to care about the little things when you had friends over. Now you think it's perfectly acceptable to do stuff like ask your guests to 'just pop the bin and recycling out when you leave'. (It's not.)

What you can do instead: Make life simpler when you're time poor. Decant a ready meal into a ceramic dish or make a one-pot comfort meal that can just bubble away. Use the extra time to tidy up (and take out the bins).

Accept your new limits.
You can't do it all.

Make your *peace* with that.

(You're still a
lovely human being.)

ON THIS DAY

DATE:

If someone doesn't understand you, that's *their* issue. Not yours.

MY NOTES
(WHAT I LOVED, FELT, WISHED, NEEDED, STRUGGLED WITH, OVERCAME)

....
....
....
....
....
....

TO DO LIST

❑ ....
❑ ....
❑ ....
❑ ....
❑ ....

THINGS TO REMEMBER
(THAT I'LL PROBABLY STILL FORGET)

....
....
....
....
....

HOW I CAN BE 'ON IT'
(WAYS TO BE A BIT MORE ORGANISED)

....
....
....
....
....

FUNNY THINGS YOU DID/SAID
(THANKS FOR MAKING ME LAUGH)

....
....
....
....
....
....
....
....
....
....
....
....
....

WHAT I WANT YOU TO KNOW
(YEARS FROM NOW)

....
....
....
....
....
....
....
....
....
....
....
....

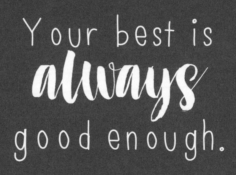

Your best is
always
good enough.

(It's your 'best' right now.
So how can it be anything less?)

ON THIS DAY

DATE:

There's only so much time. Use it wisely (and forget stuff that doesn't *really* matter).

MY NOTES
(WHAT I LOVED, FELT, WISHED, NEEDED, STRUGGLED WITH, OVERCAME)

....

....

....

....

....

....

....

....

....

....

....

....

TO DO LIST

❑ ....

❑ ....

❑ ....

❑ ....

❑ ....

GIRLS WILL BE GIRLS AND BOYS WILL BE BOYS?

KIDS ARE KIDS

After two girls, navigating the world of willies with the third came as something of a surprise and I'm often asked if I've noticed a difference between girls and boys. Sometimes, I have. Sometimes, I haven't. I was certainly not prepared for how much boys like their willies. The minute those nappies or pants come off, down goes the hand. It's like a reunion between long lost friends. Every single time. But in our gender-obsessed society, where it's no longer cool to distinguish between the sexes, where we're encouraged not to associate girls with pink and baby dolls or label boys by dressing them in blue and giving them *only* trucks, I've mostly felt that my kids are kids. End of. They're navigating their own way and making their own choices based on their desires. One of my girls is as pink as they come and has, at last count, fourteen babies (thankfully not real ones). My other has never cared much for dolls, prams or ballet. Both ride their bikes at a speed that makes my eyes water and they LOVE getting dirty. My boy hovers all over the place. He spent his first three years in his sister's pink, glittery boots but, more recently, he only wants to dress up as a pirate and collect sticks. I don't feel I've guided them in any one direction and I see, every day, that they are perfectly capable of deciding this stuff for themselves, without me sticking my nose in. I think our role is to be the backdrop to supporting their development, in whatever direction they choose. I'm not going to make a point, either way.

SMALL DIFFERENCES

That said, I *have* noticed some small behavioural differences. My boy is *so* happy for me to do stuff for him. 'Dress me, feed me, carry me...' He can do a lot of this himself but it's so much more fun making me do it. My girls, on the other hand, have always been fiercely independent, which is pretty much why they look like extras out of *Oliver!* most days. And whilst my girls love me (although some days, I'm not so sure), my boy loves me with an intensity that is sometimes overwhelming and leaves me wishing for just a smidgen of personal space. But those chubby arms around the neck? Those adoring eyes? The constant declarations of love? He knows how to woo me (which may of course be his very own form of manipulation – that the girls have mastered so well – to get me to do all the *other* stuff). I don't so much see the 'simpler' side that some say boys have; he can be as emotionally complex and needy as his sisters. Perhaps it's an effect of growing up in a female-dominated environment, where there's much drama, but I often hear my boy telling his sisters (with accompanying hands on hips), 'You've made me feel upset now, I'm not playing with you until you stop being rude to me.' So I think this is one instance where it makes a lot of sense to move beyond gender stereotypes such as, 'boys don't cry' and 'be a big, brave boy'. Supporting boys emotionally is something that we need to do and do well. *At least* as well as we naturally attempt to do it with girls.

NICE GIRLS COLOUR QUIETLY

One of the biggest myths is this one: that all girls sit around colouring quietly whilst all boys race around the house tearing it up. Some do, but many don't. Mums of boisterous boys have occasionally said to me with a wistful look in their eye, 'It must be so nice to have girls who sit quietly in the corner colouring.' I couldn't say, I've never had them. Now, at ages six and nine, they do colour nicely (and within the lines) but when they were small they could be as boisterous as any boy. I felt cheated and got really fed up of questioning myself because they *didn't* fit this profile. Likewise, I had friends with boys who thought they were over-sensitive because they *did* sit quietly and colour (and hadn't ripped out the toilet). We all worried equally, and for no reason whatsoever. Then we had more kids and realised that they're all beautifully unique and are dictated by their personalities way more than the mere presence of a penis or vagina. Ditch any unhelpful stereotypes now.

BOYS DON'T WEAR GLITTERY SHOES

Oh yes, they do. My boy has a really strong draw to anything with a heel. After his sister's pink, glittery boots came the red and white polka dot Spanish tap shoes. We've lost one but he still insists on hobbling about in the remaining one. We'd always get glances and comments when he wore them out and about, a sign that our 'progressive' world still isn't all that forward-thinking, really. It has honestly never bothered me. Why would it? I mean, who doesn't feel better able to tackle the day in a pair of pink, glittery boots? Yet, I know this is worrying for many – to find boys wearing a Disney princess dress with matching heels. I personally couldn't care less if my boy is still donning the pink boots at 18, but he probably won't be. Pretty much every one of my friends' boys have been through the same phase before turning their backs on pink and refusing to take their football strips off. Ever.

IN CONCLUSION

Sometimes, girls will be girls and boys will be boys. Other times, they won't. And that's exactly the way it should be. I'm not sure we're helping by focusing so much on gender, either way. I sometimes wonder if we draw more attention to the differences by the very act of trying *not* to accentuate them. I think we should just let kids be kids; that we shouldn't pass on inherited hang-ups from a world that is trying to be more accepting of all. That we should focus instead on *always* allowing them to feel confident about what they're doing *right now*, whilst celebrating their wonderful uniqueness and freedom of spirit to do whatever feels good, without hesitation. Because going after 'feeling good' is something we lose and something we almost don't believe we deserve the older we become. We question our happiness at every given turn and ask ourselves if it's 'right' rather than just accepting it is. So let's help our kids hang on to this very natural ability. One thing I'm totally sure of? The world would be a happier place if more people who wanted to wear glittery shoes just got those sparkly heels on.

Ditch ANY UNHELPFUL STEREOTYPES AND WATCH YOUR CHILD IN AWE FOR THE WONDERFUL, *unique* BEING THEY ARE.

(You can learn a lot from them.)

ON THIS DAY

DATE: _____

Kids never doubt
their right
to be happy.
So why should we?

MY NOTES
(WHAT I LOVED, FELT, WISHED, NEEDED, STRUGGLED WITH, OVERCAME)

....
....
....
....
....
....
....
....

TO DO LIST

☐ ....
☐ ....
☐ ....
☐ ....
☐ ....

THINGS TO REMEMBER
(THAT I'LL PROBABLY STILL FORGET)

....
....
....
....
....

WHAT MAKES YOU UNIQUE
(NEVER STOP BEING YOU)

....
....
....
....
....

FUNNY THINGS YOU DID/SAID
(THANKS FOR MAKING ME LAUGH)

....
....
....
....
....
....
....
....
....
....
....
....
....

WHAT I WANT YOU TO KNOW
(YEARS FROM NOW)

....
....
....
....
....
....
....
....
....
....
....
....
....

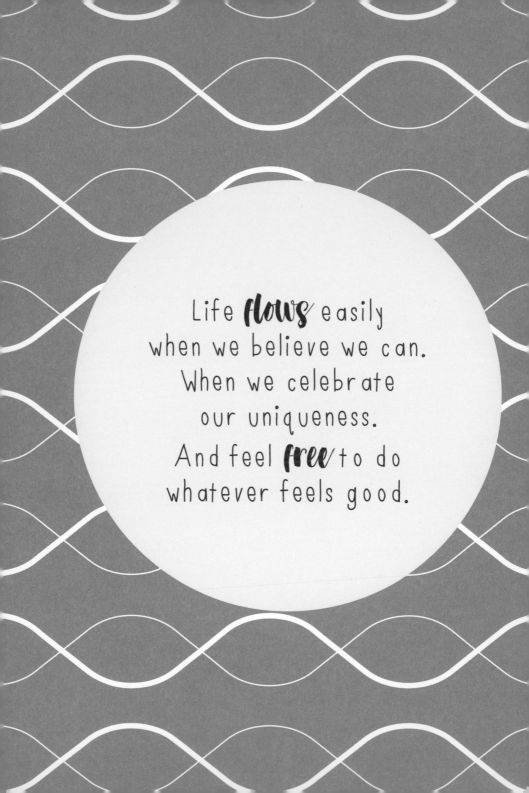

Life *flows* easily
when we believe we can.
When we celebrate
our uniqueness.
And feel *free* to do
whatever feels good.

ON THIS DAY

DATE: _____

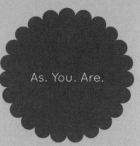

As. You. Are.

MY NOTES
(WHAT I LOVED, FELT, WISHED, NEEDED, STRUGGLED WITH, OVERCAME)

....

....

....

....

....

....

....

....

TO DO LIST

☐ ....

☐ ....

....

☐ ....

....

☐ ....

....

☐ ....

....

HAVING MORE KIDS (OR NOT)

TRYING AGAIN IS NO ONE ELSE'S BUSINESS

The decision to have more kids (and when to try to have them) is a very personal one, although you wouldn't always think so. Once your child hits the 18-month to 2-year mark, it seems to be permissible for others to ask you if/when you're having more. You might a) not have made your mind up; b) not be planning on having any more; or c) already be trying (and perhaps having more difficulty this time around). Whatever your scenario, it's totally ok to dodge this question, like you possibly did first time around when people asked, 'So *when* are you going to have children?' Suitable reactions include a) totally ignoring them; b) pointing out your current, slightly feral example of procreation (that says it all, right?); and c) changing the subject to something equally uncomfortable. Remember, you never have to explain yourself. So, if you don't want to, then don't.

'ONLY CHILDREN' ROCK

If you've decided that you're stopping at one child and are happy with your choice, good for you. There are probably a lot of parents out there who, on a challenging day, wish they'd had the good sense to do the same. If, however, you're 100% sure you don't want any more, but somehow still find yourself sitting on the fence because you've taken on board someone else's (inaccurate) comments about 'only children', stop right there. There are *many* benefits to having one child and it totally suits some parents' personalities, circumstances and goals to stop at one. Only children do not need to be spoiled or lack social skills. Some of the nicest and kindest kids I know are only children, with a perfectly balanced awareness of others. (Often, better than my own.) Also, whether you have one or five kids, first-borns tend to think they have the monopoly, any-way. And at least if you stop at one, you'll never have to listen to your eldest lament dramatically, 'My life's been SO hard since they came along', while giving their younger siblings the death stare.

WHEN CONCEIVING AGAIN IS HARD

One of the hardest things about wanting to have more kids is when it just doesn't seem to be happening. Maybe you had trouble the first time around, and it's proving difficult again. Or maybe the first time you conceived just by looking at your partner but, this time, you've been trying for months and still nothing. This can be a real shock, fill you both with uncertainty and create tension. Secondary infertility affects roughly one in seven couples and is actually more common than not being able to conceive in the first place. If you're still struggling after a year, go and see your GP who can refer you both for tests. Sometimes, these tests are inconclusive and don't highlight anything wrong with either of you. This is one of the saddest and most frustrating things for couples to bear but there are options, such as IVF. Also, 15% of couples with unexplained infertility *will* go on to conceive within a year and 35% of couples will within two years. So don't give up hope. If so much time passes that the chances of having another baby passes too, it is absolutely ok (and very important) to grieve the child you never had. It can be devastating. Life doesn't always turn out the way we hope and there's never any guilt to be had in acknowledging that. It doesn't matter if you already have a healthy child, if you wanted more, you wanted more, and you deserve to allow yourself time to make your peace with that.

HAPPY ACCIDENTS

Sometimes, babies come along when we least expect them. Particularly when you might have been using contraception, erm, creatively, or not at all (good old withdrawal – I think ten babies from within my NCT group were the result of this marvellous method. Ahem). Or perhaps you got a bit drunk and created a life after twelve pints, four bottles of wine and ten Jagermeisters (something many of us have done: no judgement here). If you had a 5-year plan, having an unplanned baby can really throw you. Especially if you're worried about money, how your partner will react (although it *does* take two to tango) or have only recently gone back to work after maternity leave. If you decide to go ahead with the pregnancy, you absolutely *will* manage and probably be all the mellower and more flexible for your little surprise. If it's a baby you didn't ever plan to have – like a third or a fourth – it can feel pretty disastrous when you first find out, even if in the end it's good news. Always take time to process what's happened. Talk to another mum with a big family who inspires you. Don't over-think the next nine months and beyond. One. Day. At a time. Go with however you're feeling and no guilt, please, for not welcoming the news with open arms. This has absolutely no bearing on the love you have, and will have, for your child. It's ok to feel like it's the end of the world for a bit (even though you'll soon see it's not). In my experience, accidental babies are the very loveliest, life-changing of blessings, once the shock has worn off. But this isn't the case for everyone – we're all different – and if you make the difficult decision not to go ahead with an unplanned pregnancy, this is no one's business but yours and your partner's (just make sure you talk to someone, should you need to). We never really have control over Mother Nature; we just like to think we do.

COPING WITH A NEWBORN AND OTHER CHILDREN

I remember the first day I was left alone with two children; a 2-week-old and a 2-year-old. I cried because their naps obviously didn't coordinate and I couldn't find time to unload the dishwasher, let alone a moment for myself. First world problems, I know. Becoming a mother of two, three, four (and so it goes on) can be HARD. Some take it in their stride, others (me) not so much. On both occasions, I found the leap to suddenly having more children tricky, and it's why I say, 'You're a new mum, no matter what round you're on.' There's some sort of illogical rationale that because you've done this motherhood lark before that you're an expert and that each time you do it again will be easier, less shocking, a walk in the park. I'm not sure, exactly, how having multiple children is supposed to make it easier. You can't just melt into the sofa and give in to the tiredness as the day plods on. There'll be a toddler having the time of his life making toilet-roll soup in the sink if you do, although at that point in the day you'll probably just be pleased that someone's taken the initiative to make any sort of meal. It's ok if, when your new arrival comes, you don't particularly feel like you're acing it. You don't have to be brilliant at it just because you've 'done it before'. I can name ten things off the top of my head that I'm still not good at, despite doing them a million times. Motherhood is no different. Every baby is new. Every time is new. The demands on you will be new. So afford yourself the same kindness you hopefully did the first time around and grab yourself a cuppa, a slab of cake and repeat after me: 'I'm a new mum, no matter what round I'm on.' (Just mind the toilet-roll soup.)

IS THREE THE MAGIC NUMBER?

Deciding whether to have a third child is one of the hardest decisions couples face unless they're a) 100% up for it; b) categorically repulsed by the idea; or c) life just feels too easy. Becoming a mum of three is the best thing I ever did, despite all the challenges it has brought with it. My thinking on having that magic third is this: go for it if one of you is up for it and the other isn't totally adverse. If you're already embracing the mammoth chaos that two kids brings. If you're happier taking a risk than possibly living a regret. If you have a niggle that there should be three, then perhaps there could be/should be three. Give it a go. Whatever you do, don't over-think it, because it's not a decision that becomes easier through debate, or which gradually makes more sense. It's one that just gets scarier, and seems even more bonkers. Instead, consider it a choice based on love, love that you already have for your two children and that you want to share with another child. Because love is often irrational, the catalyst that makes you do what's in your heart rather than what's in your head. That makes you ignore the question, 'Can I give them the most of everything?' Well, you'll already have given them the 'most' because you'll have given them each other. So, YES. If you have a nagging niggle and your partner is willing, you should totally have a third child. Because, honestly? It's utterly brilliant. (Apart from the times when it's really, really crap.)

ONE THING I LOVE ABOUT MY FAMILY:

....

....

....

....

....

HOW YOU KNOW
you're done
HAVING KIDS

There are a few signs that suggest you're over having kids:

1. **You eBay the moses basket** with the baby still in it.

2. **The thought** of laying off Pinot Grigio for another 9-plus months... well, let's not even go there.

3. **You know** that the time has finally come to do other stuff, such as build a Fortune 500 business (and drink Pinot Grigio).

4. **You've just bought a new pair of trainers.** They're neon. And pretty. And you really are going to run in them this time.

5. **The sound** of a newborn crying brings out the same reaction as that *Tubular Bells* music from *The Exorcist*.

6. **Your other half** says they would leave you. ('Not if I get there first,' you think.)

7. **Your head says no.** Your heart agrees. And your body says NO EFFING WAY!

8. **You can't bear** the thought of another 8 years at the nursery or school gates; people get less for manslaughter.

9. **Instead** of putting a 'NO JUNK MAIL' sign on your letterbox, you've put up a 'NO MORE BABIES' banner, just in case the stork has any ideas about a surprise delivery.

10. **You're on the pill.** Have a coil. And you're practising celibacy. Just to be 100 per cent sure.

11. **You have another 317 reasons** you could add to this list. Most of which involve Pinot Grigio. And sleep.

12. **Finally,** you look at your perfectly imperfect family and just know that everyone who's meant to be there, is.

your family

however it turns out
is special and loved
and uniquely yours.

(Even if it's different
to what you'd planned.)

ON THIS DAY

DATE: _____

Everything for a reason. Even if the reason isn't immediately clear.

MY NOTES
(WHAT I LOVED, FELT, WISHED, NEEDED, STRUGGLED WITH, OVERCAME)

....

....

....

....

....

....

....

....

....

....

....

TO DO LIST

☐ ....

☐ ....

☐ ....

☐ ....

☐ ....

THINGS TO REMEMBER
(THAT I'LL PROBABLY STILL FORGET)

....
....
....
....
....

MY FAMILY PLAN
(WHAT I THOUGHT IT WOULD LOOK LIKE)

....
....
....
....
....

FUNNY THINGS YOU DID/SAID
(THANKS FOR MAKING ME LAUGH)

....
....
....
....
....
....
....
....
....
....
....
....

WHAT I WANT YOU TO KNOW
(YEARS FROM NOW)

....
....
....
....
....
....
....
....
....
....
....
....

SOMETIMES
OTHER PEOPLE *sow* SEEDS
WE NEVER WISHED TO GROW.

(Always plant *your* flowers,
not someone else's weeds.)

ON THIS DAY

DATE: _____

The only person who needs to be comfortable with your decisions is YOU.

MY NOTES
(WHAT I LOVED, FELT, WISHED, NEEDED, STRUGGLED WITH, OVERCAME)

....

....

....

....

....

....

....

....

....

....

....

TO DO LIST

❏ ....

❏ ....

❏ ....

❏ ....

❏ ....

MISCARRIAGE IS HEARTBREAKING (NO MATTER WHAT)

IT IS A REALLY SAD TIME

I'm so very sorry if you're reading this having had a miscarriage. I hope that you are doing ok. I know that the sense of loss is huge. It feels like you will never recover and that the longing will never go away. Whilst miscarriage affects one in six pregnancies, this doesn't make it any easier to bear for those of us who go through it. The moment we're pregnant, we think about this new life, even when we think we aren't thinking about it at all. There are so many hopes and dreams for the future. When miscarriage takes that away from us, suddenly the calendar year stretches endlessly ahead with empty milestones we will try not to acknowledge. Losing your baby is the saddest of times. No matter how many weeks you were. No matter how many healthy kids you already have. No matter. It's really, really sad. Feel it. Share the pain, if you can. Rest and grieve. You *will* recover, but it takes time.

YOU HAVE THE RIGHT TO GRIEVE (AND YOU MUST)

Mourning your miscarriage is so important. I can't emphasise this enough. I didn't deal with mine after miscarrying our unplanned third child at work. I had just returned from maternity leave and I didn't want anyone to think I was trying for another baby, because we weren't. So I kept quiet. I carried on as normal. Going to work. Doing the nursery run. I felt desperately sad *all* of the time, but I didn't speak to anyone about it, because I just didn't know how to. Looking back, I realise I didn't think I had the right to grieve. An unplanned third baby I hadn't even decided I wanted? Two healthy kids? What did *I* have to complain about, really? It was a foolish move, on my part, because *everyone* deserves to grieve the loss of their baby, regardless of their circumstances. It is an emotional loss but also a very physical one and you should take some time out to allow your body to recover and your mind to begin to process what has happened. I wish I had done that. It took a generic letter from the health visitor, some weeks later, with the words, 'please accept our condolences,' to make me acknowledge my miscarriage and realise that of course I was 'allowed' to be sad about it. A miscarriage is never over. Just like that. And nor should it ever be.

IT DOESN'T MATTER HOW MANY KIDS YOU ALREADY HAVE

So you have one, two or three healthy children already. This doesn't mean losing a subsequent baby will not hurt. It most likely will. I remember saying to the sonographer who discovered my blighted ovum (empty sac), 'It's ok. I have two healthy girls already.' At the time, I believed my own mantra but, as it turned out, those two healthy girls made no difference whatsoever to how low I felt. In fact, they may have made it harder because I knew *exactly* what I was losing.

LET YOUR OTHER HALF IN

Miscarriage can be difficult for our other halves. They don't always know what to say if we withdraw into ourselves. When their words, flowers and cups of tea just don't touch the edge of our grief. It's really common for women to just want to be on their own and this can make a partner feel redundant and helpless. You have *both* suffered a loss, so, if you can and your partner is willing, let them in. Talk about how you feel. Ask how *they* feel. Get through your grief together. If your partner isn't understanding about how difficult this is for you, that perception of their dismissal can be really isolating. It might be that they are finding it hard themselves or that they just want to try to get back to normal. To get *you* back to normal. Tell them it's going to take time and you need their support. Don't let it become a distance between you.

OTHER PEOPLE SAY SILLY THINGS

Other people sometimes say 'silly' things when they hear about a miscarriage. 'You can try again'. 'At least it wasn't really a baby, yet'. 'You're lucky, you already have a child'. Any of these things (and more) will make you want to a) cry; b) SCREAM at them; c) use your entire arsenal of expletives. STEP BACK. Your sadness is raw. You're possibly not ready to talk about this with them yet. You might never be. They don't mean to be insensitive, they just feel they should say something and they haven't had a moment to think about what that should be. In my experience, an 'I'm so sorry' and a sincere hug is all you need to know that someone understands your pain and they're there for you.

TRY AGAIN WHEN YOU'RE READY

Some people say that you don't get over a miscarriage until you have another baby. This was certainly true for me. My planned third baby was the only thing that truly helped me heal and move on from the loss, although we did wait six months. Trying again is a really personal decision. Whilst it's recommended that you wait until after your first period post-miscarriage, the 'perfect' time is whenever *you're* ready. It's never too soon or too late, if it feels right for you. Also, it's ok to feel scared about doing it, to worry that another miscarriage will occur. Keep perspective. Because, actually, 'only' 1 per cent of women have a second miscarriage in a row, so the chances of it happening again are small. If it takes time to conceive after miscarriage, this can be agonising. Try to relax (easier said than done, I know) and send those positive vibes out into the universe. Trust that your baby is coming. Sadly, there are those who, in the end, don't get another chance and who don't get to recover from their miscarriage with another baby. Mourning your lost baby and the baby you aren't able to have is something you might need to do with a little professional help. A counsellor can help you process your feelings and give you some invaluable coping mechanisms.

For more information on counselling and to find a local counsellor, visit the MIND website: www.mind.org.uk

Everyone deserves
to grieve loss.
Whatever that
loss may be.

ON THIS DAY

DATE: _____

Feel whatever you're feeling. Always. It's the way to heal your heart.

MY NOTES
(WHAT I LOVED, FELT, WISHED, NEEDED, STRUGGLED WITH, OVERCAME)

....

....

....

....

....

....

....

....

....

....

....

TO DO LIST

❏ ....

❏ ....

❏ ....

❏ ....

❏ ....

THINGS TO REMEMBER
(THAT I'LL PROBABLY STILL FORGET)

....

....

....

....

....

MY SELF-CARE PLAN
(FOR SAD AND HARD TIMES)

....

....

....

....

....

FUNNY THINGS YOU DID/SAID
(THANKS FOR MAKING ME LAUGH)

....

....

....

....

....

....

....

....

....

....

....

....

....

WHAT I WANT YOU TO KNOW
(YEARS FROM NOW)

....

....

....

....

....

....

....

....

....

....

....

....

....

we have your back.

(You are never alone, promise.)

ON THIS DAY

DATE: _____

You will get through the tough times. You always have done.

MY NOTES
(WHAT I LOVED, FELT, WISHED, NEEDED, STRUGGLED WITH, OVERCAME)

....

....

....

....

....

....

....

TO DO LIST

.... ❑ ....

.... ❑ ....

.... ❑ ....

.... ❑ ....

.... ❑ ....

US MUMS ARE AN ARMY (CALL IN THE TROOPS)

MOTHERHOOD CAN BE LONELY

Feeling lonely as a mum isn't restricted to having a new baby, but also when feeding patterns, routines and sheer tiredness sometimes make it difficult to get out and about or to string a sentence together. Loneliness in motherhood is something that comes and goes. It often hits without much warning but, rest assured, it's perfectly normal and we all feel it, regardless of how popular we thought (hoped) we were. A lot of the loneliness is down to the constantly changing nature of motherhood and the fact that these many different phases bring mum friends into your life then take them away again. Perhaps you go back to work, your child starts preschool or your daily routine suddenly no longer fits alongside the other mums you were hanging out with. You can feel a bit lost, without the tribe you have come to rely on. They're still there, though, you may just need to try a bit harder to catch up. Also, for every phase you enter there's always a new community of mums awaiting you, if you're not afraid to open up and put yourself out there.

THE POWER OF MUM FRIENDS

Mum friends are the most powerful allies you will ever have. Simply because they get it. They understand your life – the joys, challenges and frustrations – without you having to say a thing. When you're dawdling (painfully) down the road to buy a loaf of bread with a toddler in tow, who insists on examining that teeny, tiny crack in the pavement, *they know*. When your heart is breaking because you're leaving your child sobbing at nursery again, that hand on your shoulder immediately tells you *they know*. When you're worried about your child's behaviour or your relationship with your partner, they listen without judgement, because *they know*. And when you're in trouble, a mum friend will (hopefully) step up to help where she can, no questions asked. Simply because she gets it.

IF YOU DON'T SAY, THEY DON'T KNOW

Sometimes, however, we don't give others an opportunity to help us when we're navigating stormy seas. We power on when things *aren't* fine and we don't tell our allies, like we once might have. Not because we're trying to put on a brave face or because we don't want to share it with anyone, but purely because we didn't have a chance or we hadn't realised that things had got on top of us. Suddenly, the tiredness has caught up or a tricky situation threatens to momentarily overwhelm us. Engulfed in that moment, we feel marooned, forgotten and left out. We wonder why no one has noticed we're struggling, choosing to ignore the fact that we've only just seen it ourselves. It seems like everyone else has their s*** together and they're all so happy and in harmony with one another. The truth is that everyone is waging their own daily battles, no matter how small, and no one has it together *all* of the time. But when we become disconnected from one another, or forget to check in with each other, we aren't able to see this and we lose the chance to be supported and to support others.

CALL IN THE TROOPS

None of us are mind-readers, although mum friends can be pretty close sometimes. But amidst the busy lives we all lead and the frequently stressful mornings just trying to get out of the house, it's impossible to expect to be in tune with one another all of the time. So, if you're struggling, TELL SOMEONE. Pick up the phone. Drop a friend a text. Meet for a coffee. You'll feel way better for talking things through and for making that connection again. Also, what I've always found is that any mum friend you call will be as grateful as you are for the opportunity to chat, because they are often struggling too or feeling a bit lost. And guess what? They also thought you (and everyone else) had their s*** together. Mum friends step up when they're asked. They care that you're having a tough time. And when they're aware, they'll do whatever they can to help. Because us mums are an army. And we leave no mum behind.

ON THIS DAY

DATE: _____

You always have the opportunity to make someone else feel better. Take it.

MY NOTES
(WHAT I LOVED, FELT, WISHED, NEEDED, STRUGGLED WITH, OVERCAME)

....

....

....

....

....

....

....

....

....

....

....

TO DO LIST

❑ ....

❑ ....

❑ ....

❑ ....

❑ ....

THINGS TO REMEMBER
(THAT I'LL PROBABLY STILL FORGET)

....
....
....
....
....

FRIENDS I CAN CALL
(WHO ALWAYS LOVE TO HELP)

....
....
....
....
....

FUNNY THINGS YOU DID/SAID
(THANKS FOR MAKING ME LAUGH)

....
....
....
....
....
....
....
....
....
....
....
....
....

WHAT I WANT YOU TO KNOW
(YEARS FROM NOW)

....
....
....
....
....
....
....
....
....
....
....
....
....

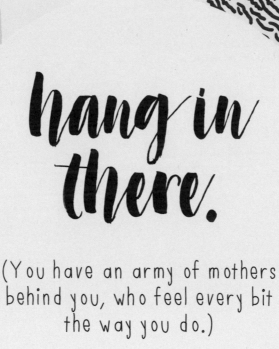

hang in there.

(You have an army of mothers behind you, who feel every bit the way you do.)

ON THIS DAY

DATE: _____

MY NOTES
(WHAT I LOVED, FELT, WISHED, NEEDED, STRUGGLED WITH, OVERCAME)

....

....

....

....

....

....

....

....

....

....

....

....

TO DO LIST

☐ ....

☐ ....

☐ ....

☐ ....

☐ ....

TWO-IN-ONE SLOW-COOKED SPAGHETTI BOLOGNESE AND LASAGNE

Lasagne can feel like such a faff to make. But if you make a spaghetti bolognese then keep back a bit of meat, you've only got to make the cheese sauce and you can assemble one in minutes. Two dinners. Just like that. The grated carrot is optional, but it adds some secret veg, as do the mushrooms, unless your child thinks they're the actual spawn of The Slug Devil, as mine clearly do.

BOLOGNESE SAUCE
Half a portion serves 4
(2 adults and 2 kids)

INGREDIENTS
Glug of olive oil
1 crushed/chopped garlic clove
1 chopped onion
750g minced beef
400g chopped tomatoes/passata
Generous squirt of tomato puree
1 carrot, grated (optional)
Handful of quartered mushrooms (optional)
Spaghetti
(50g per child, 100g per adult)
Grated cheese to serve (optional)

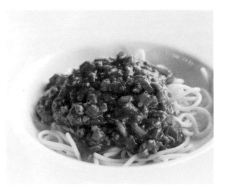

METHOD
Heat the oil in a pan and fry the garlic and onion until soft. After a few minutes make a large well in the veg, then add the mince and cook until it is browned. Stir in the tomatoes, puree and carrot (optional) and leave to simmer for 25 minutes. After this time, add the mushrooms, if you're using them, and cook for a few minutes until softened. Once cooked, set half of the sauce aside for your lasagne. Serve the other half with some spaghetti, cooked as per the packet instructions. Top with grated cheese.

LASAGNE

Serves 4 (2 adults and 2 kids)

INGREDIENTS

Bolognese sauce portion
(opposite)
8–12 lasagne sheets
Cheese sauce (below)

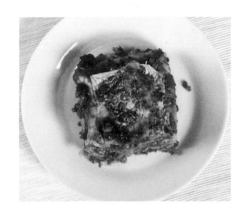

EASY PEASY CHEESE SAUCE

50g butter
50g flour
300ml milk
1 tablespoon soft cheese
(optional)
50g grated cheese

METHOD

To make the cheese sauce, melt the butter in a pan, then add the flour and cook it off for a minute or two, stirring constantly. Add the milk and whisk continually over a low heat until it starts to thicken. Once it's taken on the consistency of a sauce, remove from the heat and add the soft and grated cheese and stir until melted. Simple!

To assemble the lasagne, you'll need a baking dish. Make do with whatever you have! I've used a rectangular dish before and just filled three-quarters of it. Preheat your oven to 180°C/Gas Mark 4. Lay a thin layer of bolognese over the bottom of the dish, drizzle with the cheese sauce and put 4–6 lasagne sheets on top. Repeat. Cover the last layer of lasagne fully with the cheese sauce, grate some more cheese on top and put in the oven for 35–40 minutes. Serve with garlic bread and salad or cucumber and carrot sticks.

ON THIS DAY

DATE: _____

No one gets it like another mum. They SEE you.

MY NOTES
(WHAT I LOVED, FELT, WISHED, NEEDED, STRUGGLED WITH, OVERCAME)

....

....

....

....

....

....

....

....

....

....

....

TO DO LIST

☐ ....

☐ ....

☐ ....

☐ ....

☐ ....

THINGS TO REMEMBER
(THAT I'LL PROBABLY STILL FORGET)

....
....
....
....
....

OTHER RECIPES YOU LIKE
(HURRAH FOR THAT!)

....
....
....
....
....

FUNNY THINGS YOU DID/SAID
(THANKS FOR MAKING ME LAUGH)

....
....
....
....
....
....
....
....
....
....
....
....
....

WHAT I WANT YOU TO KNOW
(YEARS FROM NOW)

....
....
....
....
....
....
....
....
....
....
....

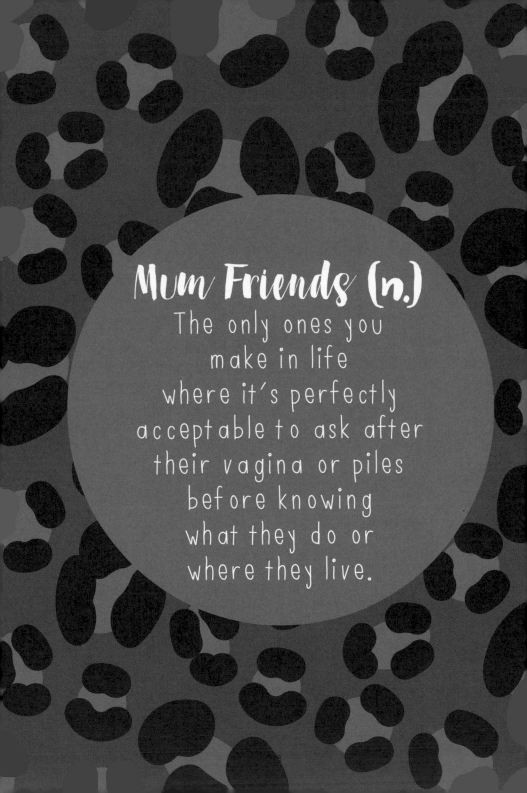

Mum Friends (n.)
The only ones you
make in life
where it's perfectly
acceptable to ask after
their vagina or piles
before knowing
what they do or
where they live.

ON THIS DAY

DATE: _____

Opening up is the greatest gift we can give each other.

MY NOTES
(WHAT I LOVED, FELT, WISHED, NEEDED, STRUGGLED WITH, OVERCAME)

....

....

....

....

....

....

....

....

....

....

TO DO LIST

❏ ....

❏ ....

❏ ....

❏ ....

❏ ....

THE NOT-SO-NEW MUM'S F*CKET LIST

Here's a list of things that are perfectly reasonable to let go when you're raising kids, which you can use as a handy guide until they leave home (and maybe even beyond...).

1. **Always being on time for stuff.** My dad once told me a marvellous saying: 'You should never be early, because you're wasting your time, and you should never be late, because then you're wasting someone else's.' I've always loved this. However, since three kids entered my life, I have a new saying: 'I've got kids. And I have no idea if I'll turn up on time. Or, in fact, at all.' It's taken me a while to get my head around the fact that we're so often late, and to not feel bad about it. Because whilst us mums might do everything in our power to be on time, the truth is we have unpredictable small people in our care who frequently screw that up. It's NOT our fault. It's not.

2. **Being a good hostess.** I always feel slightly apologetic when we invite people over, especially if they don't have kids. In the privacy of our own home I know that we are chaotic, but there's something about doing it in front of an audience that REALLY makes you see this. I'll also never forgive myself for thinking it's acceptable to ask my guests to do stuff like replace the toilet roll, 'whilst they're up there'. But you know what? It's entertaining, if nothing else, and no one really expects us to be domestic goddesses. So accept your limitations, pull open a few bags of posh crisps and grab the 'special occasion' bottle from the back of the fridge. Because what's the one really good thing about dining with parents? We ALWAYS have plenty of booze.

3. **Being calm.** I'm not even going to elaborate on this one. I'm simply going to say, it's ok to shout. And to say FFS under your breath (loudly) 457 times a day.

4. **Taking on board other people's s***.** Us mums used to be fairly tolerant souls, I think. These days? Not so much. Our patience is already tested to the max by small people who we actually love. People who we aren't so keen on or we don't even know? We ain't got no time for their rubbish. And that's ok. (Save your energy for the ones that matter.)

220

5. **Being on top of stuff.** Once your child starts nursery, it feels like there is so much to keep on top of: dressing-up days, contact books, permission slips to go to the sodding park. Arghhhhhhh! So forgive yourself if, like me, you forget most of it. You are only one woman and you can only remember so much. And, let's face it, if your kid's actual name often proves tricky to keep a hold of, you haven't got a hope in hell with the other stuff. Make your peace with that now. And move on.

6. **Being rational.** It's really hard to be rational when you're tired and emotionally and physically stretched. Always make allowances for yourself when you feel like this. And take it as a warning sign that you need a bit of TLC.

7. **Being perfect at anything (especially motherhood).** I used to be a perfectionist. Now I'm often so worn-down that I need reminding to buy new leggings for the girls because theirs have holes in. On the other hand, us mums know that nothing *really* bad comes of wearing holey leggings. And that as long as we are all fed and safe, we're doing just fine. (Plus being a perfectionist is exhausting and not all it's cracked up to be.)

8. **Being everything to everyone.** The lack of headspace when you're a mum is CRAZY. There are a million, unrelated thoughts running through our minds at any given moment. 'What am I going to make them for dinner?' 'Bugger, did I turn the tumble dryer on?' 'When is *The Great British Bake-Off* coming back?' 'Can I move that deadline?' There is no way on this earth that we can be everything to everyone ALL of the time. So it's absolutely ok to ask for some space (and get it). Being a 'mum martyr' is not sustainable and it's fine to have someone else take over the responsibility of keeping the kids alive for a bit. We've earned it. A million unrelated thoughts over.

ON THIS DAY

DATE: _____

You WILL forget stuff. So what? You always do the stuff that matters. Eventually.

MY NOTES
(WHAT I LOVED, FELT, WISHED, NEEDED, STRUGGLED WITH, OVERCAME)

....

....

....

....

....

....

....

....

....

....

....

....

TO DO LIST

❏ ....

❏ ....

❏ ....

❏ ....

❏ ....

THINGS TO REMEMBER
(THAT I'LL PROBABLY STILL FORGET)

....

....

....

....

....

STUFF I CAN LET GO
(I DON'T NEED TO BE SUPERMUM)

....

....

....

....

....

FUNNY THINGS YOU DID/SAID
(THANKS FOR MAKING ME LAUGH)

....

....

....

....

....

....

....

....

....

....

....

....

....

WHAT I WANT YOU TO KNOW
(YEARS FROM NOW)

....

....

....

....

....

....

....

....

....

....

....

....

....

You do not
need to be
everything
to everyone.

(It's impossible. And it's
unfulfilling.)

ON THIS DAY

DATE: _____

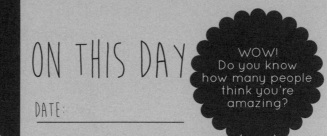

WOW!
Do you know
how many people
think you're
amazing?

MY NOTES
(WHAT I LOVED, FELT, WISHED, NEEDED, STRUGGLED WITH, OVERCAME)

....

....

....

....

....

....

....

....

TO DO LIST

❏ ....

❏ ....

❏ ....

❏ ....

❏ ....

THE TRUTH ABOUT THREENAGERS

YOU THOUGHT TODDLERS WERE BAD

And then they become a threenager. If you're reading this with one already in tow, you're probably nodding along. If you're still in toddler mode and now freaking out that there's a stage more illogical than that one, don't panic. In two short (really long) years they'll be at school and you'll miss them like crazy. Honestly.

THREENAGERS KNOW IT ALL

Threenagers aren't *really* that different to their toddler counterparts. They're still largely illogical and their behaviour can be – shall we say – demanding. But they're developing that 'Look at me, I'm cooler than you,' vibe, followed by 'I know WAY more than you, so please don't pretend you're in charge here. You're not. I know it. You know it. The manky old cat knows it.' This is the major difference. The sudden acceleration in their development – mobility and vocabulary – makes them *think* they've suddenly got the goods to back up all the other stuff. It spells INDEPENDENCE for them and TROUBLE for you. Yes, threenagers think they are cleverer than you. The End. (There is a distinct possibility that, after spending 12 hours with one, they are. Given that you have lost the will to live, several times over.)

INDEPENDENCE DAY (WITHOUT WILL SMITH)

Threenagers are ALL about doing stuff for themselves. And they're way worse than a disillusioned toddler who *thinks* they're independent, because threenagers can actually do things now. Getting in and out of the car. Putting on their own shoes. Sadly for you, they're not as good at this as they think they are. Which means you'll be even later for stuff you were never on time for anyway.

TORTURE BY TALKING

You couldn't wait for them to say their first word. You encouraged them every step of the way by pointing things out and reading that sodding *First 100 Words* book. Now? They won't shut up. Yup. Many threenagers talk. A lot. Sometimes, all day long. And you have no one to blame but yourself. Because all you've done is arm them with the skills to torment you. Every single day. For the rest of time. Arghhhhh!

WHEN THREENAGERS GET ANGRY

Angering a threenager is not something you want to do too often. They're a bit more considered than toddlers when it comes to acting up, though. Tantrums are too obvious. They'll go for something much subtler, which will completely catch you off guard and leave you unprepared for attack. Like refusing to put on their coat by sitting in uncharacteristic silence on the stairs with a face of thunder. This basically means you're screwed and you're not going to do any of the things you wanted to do, because you're just too exhausted to face battling them in order to get to the shops. Sometimes they'll throw in a 'hand on hip'. They've seen grown-ups do this rather successfully and swiftly added it to their repertoire. This is just another way of them telling you they're not doing it. Any of it.

'IT WASN'T ME'

Oh good. Another cracking development. Threenagers learn how to fib. Welcome to their disillusioned world. You saw them hit their sister over the head/throw their crisp packet on the floor/take something that isn't theirs WITH YOUR ACTUAL EYES. They swear blind it wasn't them. 'I saw you do it!' you say. Several times. They look at you with disgust. To them, YOU are the fibber. And a bad one at that. The death stare is coming your way. Any. Minute. Now. (Take cover.)

ON THIS DAY

DATE: _____

As you weather another new 'phase', remember, this one will pass too.

MY NOTES
(WHAT I LOVED, FELT, WISHED, NEEDED, STRUGGLED WITH, OVERCAME)

....

....

....

....

....

....

....

....

....

....

....

TO DO LIST

☐ ....

☐ ....

☐ ....

☐ ....

☐ ....

THINGS TO REMEMBER
(THAT I'LL PROBABLY STILL FORGET)

....

....

....

....

....

STUFF YOU CAN'T LET GO
(AND THE REASON WE'RE ALWAYS LATE)

....

....

....

....

....

FUNNY THINGS YOU DID/SAID
(THANKS FOR MAKING ME LAUGH)

....

....

....

....

....

....

....

....

....

....

....

....

WHAT I WANT YOU TO KNOW
(YEARS FROM NOW)

....

....

....

....

....

....

....

....

....

....

....

....

demanding.
HILARIOUS.
frustrating.
BEGUILING.

(Life with kids is never dull.)

ON THIS DAY

DATE: _____

Stop. And listen to what your child is saying. They could do stand-up.

MY NOTES
(WHAT I LOVED, FELT, WISHED, NEEDED, STRUGGLED WITH, OVERCAME)

....

....

....

....

....

....

....

....

....

....

....

TO DO LIST

❏ ....

❏ ....

❏ ....

❏ ....

❏ ....

HOW TO TOILET-TRAIN (WITHOUT LOSING YOUR S***)

GO WITH THE FLOW

I've toilet-trained three children now. You might think (hope) this makes me an expert with lots of useful tips. Unfortunately, it doesn't. The first time was disastrous. The second two times were better, simply because I totally winged it. And I realised something. The less interest you take in 'training' them, the easier it seems to be. Get all worked up, obsess about it, talk about it endlessly and I think, just maybe, the whole process scares the bejeezus out of our poor kids. This is one occasion where it really is advisable to go with the flow (pun intended).

WAIT UNTIL YOU'RE BOTH READY

This is the most important thing to bear in mind and has the most impact on how successful your toilet-training effort is going to be. Waiting until you're BOTH ready. You and *your* child. Not your friend and *their* child. Or your mother-in-law's friend's daughter's child who's the same age and is dry during the day AND at night. If other people are *that* keen for your child to be toilet-trained, then hand your child over to them with 271 pairs of pants and tell them to bring them home when they're done. That usually kills any interest. It's your and your child's business (pun intended again) and no one else's.

THERE'S NO RUSH

My first was just two years and three months when we started because I had another baby on the way and I had that misconception that NO WAY ON EARTH COULD I POSSIBLY HAVE TWO IN NAPPIES. It wasn't even my own misconception, but a seed sown by someone else. (I have since learned that the world doesn't actually end when you DO have two in nappies. I've done it. You just buy a few more nappies, that's all.) Anyway, she wasn't ready and neither was I. I was heavily pregnant, hormonal and generally a bit miserable and the whole experience was stressful. We had rewards, charts and incentives coming out of our ears and still she wanted to wee on the floor and poo in her pants. We did persevere and we did sort of get there in the end but she had accidents for months after and I'm pretty certain we wouldn't have had if I'd waited until we were both ready. Her sister was three when we toilet-trained. So was their brother. Both were done in a week, with pretty much a total lack of interest from me.

SOMETIMES, ALL YOU NEED IS A GIANT SWORD

When I started toilet-training my boy, everyone said it would be really different to 'doing' girls. Way harder, they said (although they hadn't been on the sidelines watching me and daughter number one). It's true there were some differences. For one, dazzling him with a variety of pants (like I once did his fashion-conscious sisters) did nothing to convince him that sitting on a potty was something he couldn't *wait* to do. In those first couple of days, he couldn't have cared less whether he was p***ing all over Superman or Batman. To be fair, it's impossible to identify the cause of his initial apathy because, being the third child, I was completely inconsistent about the whole process. Forget the reward charts and bag of goodies for each wee, there was the mention of a stale old chocolate biscuit if he did one. Which I then ate, absentmindedly. After two hours of a COMPLETE lack of interest on day one, I caved and put on a nappy. Some books will tell you this is STRICTLY FORBIDDEN AND YOU WILL GO TO HELL IF YOU DO THIS. But I simply didn't want to force him before he was ready. (Official story: I wanted to watch *Mad Men*.) Then, just when I'd resolved to try again in 2 to 3 years, he took himself off, sword in hand, sat on the potty and did a wee. And it turned out that all he actually needed was a giant cutlass. The moral of the story? Sometimes, all the will in the world (and sticker charts) doesn't achieve the end goal. Often, all you need to do is chill out, eat a stale biscuit and watch a bit of Netflix. Who knew?

NIGHTTIME BEDWETTING IS PERFECTLY NORMAL

There's a lot of focus on *when* your child is dry at night. Far too much. You can find yourself spending a lot of time thinking about this. What's normal. What's not. Why your child isn't dry at two, three, four or five when your friend's child was dry the very first night they started toilet-training. IT'S IRRELEVANT. Because it's not something you can control, in my experience. My eldest wasn't dry at night until almost seven and still has the odd accident. Yet, her sister was dry at night after a week, aged three; it had absolutely nothing to do with anything I did (or didn't) do. Because, for *many* kids, being dry at night depends on whether they are physically capable. In children under nine, it's common for their little brains to produce a low level of antidiuretic hormone (the hormone responsible for regulating fluid in the body). So when they go to sleep, the brain doesn't tell the bladder that it's full and it essentially overflows without waking the child. Nevertheless, you'll probably hear lots of schools of thought on nighttime toilet-training. Some say you should take your child's nighttime nappy away when it's been dry a few mornings running. Others say take them away regardless and then do the nighttime 'lifting', where you take your child to the toilet before you go to bed yourself. But, remember that many children aren't dry at night for years after mastering the daytime, so don't stress about it if yours isn't. Experts suggest that if your child is still regularly wetting their bed aged nine upwards, you should take them to the doctors to rule out any physical implications. Until then, I think it's better to just go with it, be patient and figure out what works best for your child (and you). One of the best lines you'll hear repeatedly in parenting *totally* applies here: 'They won't still be doing it when they're eighteen.'

There's no rush.
Do it when YOU and YOUR
child are ready.

(This mantra applies to
everything in motherhood.)

ON THIS DAY

DATE: _____

If something feels stressful, don't force it. Try again tomorrow.

MY NOTES
(WHAT I LOVED, FELT, WISHED, NEEDED, STRUGGLED WITH, OVERCAME)

....

....

....

....

....

....

....

....

....

....

....

TO DO LIST

❏ ....

❏ ....

❏ ....

❏ ....

❏ ....

THINGS TO REMEMBER
(THAT I'LL PROBABLY STILL FORGET)

....
....
....
....
....

YOUR FAVOURITE TOYS
(AND OTHER BRIBES FOR TOILET-TRAINING)

....
....
....
....
....

FUNNY THINGS YOU DID/SAID
(THANKS FOR MAKING ME LAUGH)

....
....
....
....
....
....
....
....
....
....
....
....

WHAT I WANT YOU TO KNOW
(YEARS FROM NOW)

....
....
....
....
....
....
....
....
....
....
....
....

you're doing a really

good job

(I know it doesn't
always feel that way.)

ON THIS DAY

DATE: _____

Try to parent from a good place and mindset. It will serve you way better.

MY NOTES
(WHAT I LOVED, FELT, WISHED, NEEDED, STRUGGLED WITH, OVERCAME)

....

....

....

....

....

....

....

....

....

....

....

TO DO LIST

☐ ....

☐ ....

☐ ....

☐ ....

☐ ....

NO MUM REALLY ENJOYS SOFT PLAY OR PLAYDATES (PHEW)

AS PAINFUL AS LABOUR

There are some things in motherhood that are just not meant to be enjoyed, no matter how brilliant a mum you are (and you are). Soft play and playdates are up there on that list. Oh and, just like labour, you'll repeatedly forget just how painful the experience is, until you find yourself right back there again. And again. And again. You're not alone.

SOFT PLAY IS GENIUS! (UNTIL IT'S NOT)

When you first go to soft play you think it's genius. It's enclosed. They have squishy surfaces to bolster insane toddlers and threen-agers. And they have coffee. PURE GENIUS. What you've forgotten to factor in is the forty insane toddlers and threenagers that ruin the whole experience. Your own is particularly tricky and insists on eating soggy rice cakes in the middle of the soft play equip-ment. Even though eating is STRICTLY forbidden. That's what the tables at the side are for. Obviously. When you planned this trip, you imagined that you would sit on those lovely tables at the side, drinking coffee. The reality sees you trying to squeeze your body under nets, through tiny tunnels and down slides in a bid to encour-age your child to step away from the snacks and make the most of the tenner you paid to get in there in the first place. This is why you pay £40 a month *not* to go the gym. You don't need any more vigorous exercise, thank you. If you're lucky, there will be a ball pool, which you can maroon yourself in whilst your child (and everyone else's) throws plastic balls at your head. You would not be the first mum to consider how long it would take to suffocate yourself in there.

HOW TO SURVIVE A PLAYDATE

There's only ONE way to have a successful, enjoyable playdate, and that's for the other parent to do it at *their* house. The problem with this, however, is that one playdate leads to another. So once you're on the oh so merry merry-go-round, there's no getting off. All you can then hope for is for your child to behave so hideously that you get kicked off. In the early days of motherhood, a playdate, a bit like soft play, sounds like a really lovely idea. You remember going round to your friend's house when you were small, playing in their room, eating a delicious tea and having a jolly nice time. Well, that's how *you* remember it, anyway. What you didn't see was the mother who was hosting you, pulling her hair out and counting down the minutes until you went home.

Fast-forward twenty-five or so years and it's your go. Until children turn school-age, the other parent usually stays (which can actually be a pretty nice way to spend an afternoon), but there's always the rather jaded mum of older kids who forgets this etiquette (not me, ahem) and leaves their crazy three-year-old with you ALL ALONE. And the minute the friend turns up, your child suddenly decides they'd like some quiet time in their room – which has obviously *never* happened before. What this means is that YOU are now the playdate and you'll have to haul out the pipe cleaners and create something pipe cleanery. So, not only do you hate crafts (come on, I know I'm not the only one), but now you're actually doing them with someone else's kid. Marvellous. You will also have to cook *actual* food, because you don't want to be *that* parent who serves up fish fingers and peas. Or, worse, plain pasta. So you go all out and do something wild with courgettes. And then give everyone a bag of Hula Hoops when they refuse to eat it. Don't worry, you'll soon learn and serve plain pasta forever more.

Some 2 hours later (it feels like 37), the other parent will (hopefully) collect their child and ask you how it went. And even though your child is screaming and theirs looks utterly bewildered, you will both pretend it went really well. They'll find themselves saying, 'We must do this again. I'll call you to set something up.' Whilst you nod your head manically and stick imaginary pins in your eyes. It's like a bad date from your twenties, all over again. Happy days.

ON THIS DAY

If the thought of doing 'it' fills you with dread, Just. Don't. Do. It.

DATE: _____

MY NOTES
(WHAT I LOVED, FELT, WISHED, NEEDED, STRUGGLED WITH, OVERCAME)

....

....

....

....

....

....

....

....

....

....

....

TO DO LIST

❏ ....

❏ ....

❏ ....

❏ ....

❏ ....

THINGS TO REMEMBER
(THAT I'LL PROBABLY STILL FORGET)

....

....

....

....

....

PLAYDATES TO ARRANGE
(DO I REALLY WANT TO DO THIS?)

....

....

....

....

....

FUNNY THINGS YOU DID/SAID
(THANKS FOR MAKING ME LAUGH)

....

....

....

....

....

....

....

....

....

....

....

....

....

WHAT I WANT YOU TO KNOW
(YEARS FROM NOW)

....

....

....

....

....

....

....

....

....

....

....

....

....

You don't have to enjoy
every little thing
about motherhood.

(But look for the joy
whenever you can.)

ON THIS DAY

DATE: _____

Sometimes we need to be less busy. And just 'be'.

MY NOTES
(WHAT I lOVED, FELT, WISHED, NEEDED, STRUGGLED WITH, OVERCAME)

....

....

....

....

....

....

....

....

....

....

....

TO DO LIST

❏ ....

❏ ....

❏ ....

❏ ....

❏ ....

10 LAST-MINUTE DRESSING-UP IDEAS (THEM NOT YOU)

Dressing up used to mean a nice dress and pair of heels. For you. Now it's frantically remembering it's World Book Day/Children In Need/Let's Dress Up for the Sheer Hell of It Day at 10.00 pm the night before. Arghhhh! Well, there's no need to be super organised and splash the cash. Raid the cupboards for old tablecloths, worn shirts and things you'd totally forgotten you owned and you'll be amazed at what you can come up with, when you're really up against it. Trust me, I've done it (and I'm no seamstress either). Keep procreating and, eventually, you'll have so many dressing-up outfits that you'll have to dedicate a whole wardrobe to them. Which reminds me, NEVER throw away any 'new' creation. Today's outfit is tomorrow's hand-me-down. So, without further ado, here are some easy outfits you can pull off at the eleventh hour with a bit of imagination, a needle and thread, YouTube and a Twirl.

1. Little Red Riding Hood. Quite a few of the Disney outfits come with red capes (think Snow White) but if you haven't got one, you can make one really easily out of a bit of red fabric – think redundant tablecloths – or even an old red dress (I used an old red maternity one. RIP). If you're using an old frock, you can snip it open and cut off the sleeves, attaching one of them to the back of the fabric as a hood. Complete the look with a basket of any description.

2. Veruca Salt. Easily made if your daughter already has a red dress (and an attitude). Just cut out and attach a semi-circle of white fabric for the collar (snip the middle out of the bottom so you're left with an upside-down M shape) and a couple of long rectangles for the white cuffs. Add a black belt, some white tights and black shoes. Finish off with an Alice band for the hair, and write 'I WANT IT NOW!' on a piece of paper, which you can stick to a pencil for them to hold. It doesn't matter if you don't have the exact look, do what you can!

3. Alice in Wonderland. It's surprising, when you have a rummage, how many gingham or blue-and-white stripy dresses/tops your child actually has. Or is that just mine? This is another outfit that can be mocked up with whatever you have to hand. For the apron, cut a semi-circle out of any old white fabric, leaving a long strip at the top, which can be the ties to secure it around your child's waist. Add some tights and cute Mary-Jane shoes, which you probably own anyway, and you're done!

4. Matilda. Blue dress. Red ribbon in their hair. And a (small) pile of books to carry. Done.

5. Minion. If you've got the clothing already, you just need some face paints for this one. Simply dress your child in some blue dungarees, paint their face yellow and add some swimming goggles, black gloves and black shoes. (Thanks to my girls for the inspiration for this one, when I left them decorating cakes and came back to find them turning their brother yellow with food colouring.)

6. Egyptian mummy. Not just restricted to Halloween, this one can also be used for World Book Day (fact). Put your child in dark leggings and a top. And wrap them in strips of toilet roll or actual bandages, tying every few strips so it doesn't just fall off in one dramatic exodus.

7. Charlie Brown. This one works particularly well on children with really fair/fine/no hair. Black shorts, black shoes and a yellow t-shirt with a black zig-zag, which you can either paint/draw on/or cut out from a piece of fabric and stick/sew on. Make your own placard with 'Good Grief' written on it, using the method in no. 2 (sensing a theme here?).

8. Emoji. Pick your favourite emoji. Grab an old box and cut out two big card circles to fit your child's body. Paint them yellow on one side (the circles, not your child), draw your expression on the front circle, punch a hole in the 'shoulders' of each circle, and then thread/tie string to join them up, so that your child can wear it over their head like a sandwich board. This method also works for a playing card outfit – just add a red or black design of your choice to a white rectangular background (*Alice in Wonderland* strikes again).

9. 'Anything around a combination of items you own.' This is basically why the internet was invented. For food shopping AND dressing-up days. Seriously. I have often just panicked at 7.30 that morning and typed in whatever was needed, like, 'Saints who wear red capes', for the imminent Dressing Up As A Saint Day, which I'd totally forgotten about. I've always come up trumps. Another victory for the Last-minute Mum. Either that, or the fact you'll make anything work when you're desperate enough.

10. Any pre-made Disney Princess/Spiderman costume you already have. No, this is NOT cheating. And, yes, it's perfectly ok to recycle it for every dressing-up day that comes your way. Unless they're giving out prizes and that prize is two weeks in the Caribbean, do you care, *really*?

WORLD BOOK DAY NOTE
Yes, apparently, the character *does* have to come from a book. But, in my experience (and every other parents', I've met), there's ALWAYS a book to match the character. If you look hard enough/ embellish/completely make it up. And anyway, who's to say what came first? The book or the film? It's a bit chicken and egg really, isn't it? If in doubt/hot water, make *that* your line and stick to it.

What we dressed up as before (so we don't forget):

Age 1 ....

Age 2 ....

Age 3 ....

Age 4 ....

Don't panic.
YOU'VE GOT THIS.
AND YOU WILL
SUCCEED. AGAIN.

(Because you're particularly resourceful
and brilliant at the eleventh hour.)

ON THIS DAY

DATE: _____

Never compare your effort to another mum's. We all have different strengths.

MY NOTES
(WHAT I LOVED, FELT, WISHED, NEEDED, STRUGGLED WITH, OVERCAME)

....

....

....

....

....

....

....

....

....

....

....

TO DO LIST

☐ ....

☐ ....

☐ ....

☐ ....

☐ ....

THINGS TO REMEMBER
(THAT I'LL PROBABLY STILL FORGET)

....
....
....
....
....

DRESSING-UP IDEAS
(PREFERABLY USING STUFF WE ALREADY OWN)

....
....
....
....
....

FUNNY THINGS YOU DID/SAID
(THANKS FOR MAKING ME LAUGH)

....
....
....
....
....
....
....
....
....
....
....
....
....

WHAT I WANT YOU TO KNOW
(YEARS FROM NOW)

....
....
....
....
....
....
....
....
....
....
....
....
....

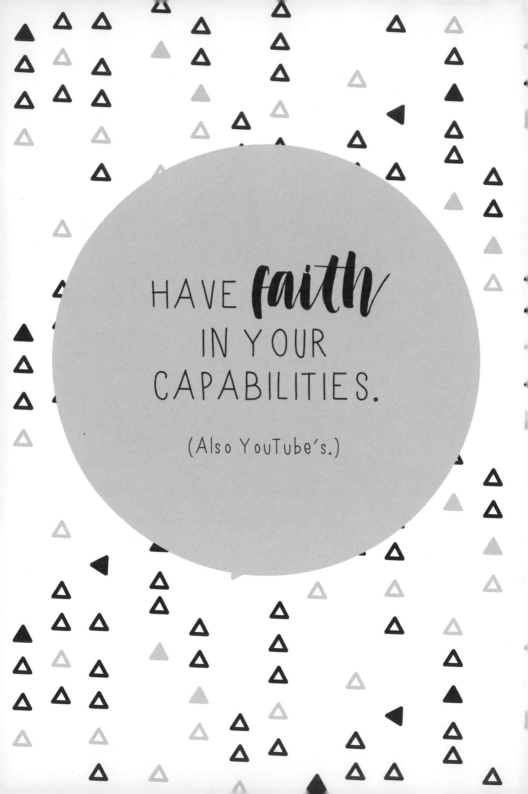

HAVE *faith*
IN YOUR
CAPABILITIES.

(Also YouTube's.)

ON THIS DAY

DATE: _____

Whatever you do, you do it with love. And that can never be anything but perfect.

MY NOTES
(WHAT I LOVED, FELT, WISHED, NEEDED, STRUGGLED WITH, OVERCAME)

....

....

....

....

....

....

....

....

....

....

....

TO DO LIST

❏ ....

❏ ....

❏ ....

❏ ....

❏ ....

LOOK AFTER YOUR MIND AND BODY

YOU FIRST

'Self-care' is such a buzz phrase these days. Too often, though, we talk about it without *really* doing it. But the days of being a martyr to motherhood are over (or, rather, they need to be). We absolutely have to learn to put ourselves first sometimes, to not feel guilty about it and get better at asking for help, especially when our children are small. Running ourselves into the ground helps no one, least of all the small people we are trying to nurture. When you look at it like that, putting yourself first is actually putting them first too. You're also showing your child that it's important to value themselves. That YOU are a person too. And that's their first lesson in self-esteem, right there.

PLEASE YOURSELF

Most of us wouldn't treat another person the way we treat ourselves. Why does everyone else get the best of us? Why do we leave ourselves with ZERO resources? Why do we so often tell ourselves we SHOULD do something? If you're telling yourself this, you probably don't want to do it anyway. Spend the time doing something you DO want to do, instead. Liberating, eh?

TAKE TIME OUT

My four-year-old is happiest when he is by my side, talking to me every second of every 13+ hour day. He also additionally sometimes likes to see me in the middle of the night to a) ask me to straighten his bedsheets; b) tell me he's never going to leave me (slightly creepy at the best of times, but at 3.00 am?); c) talk to me about pirates or whatever other urgent matter has popped into his mind. This means that there are (many) days where I feel like I am going insane. I know that this is the same for you and all mums out there. The kids need us. They want us. They get us. In my experience, there is no cure for this except time out. (Reclaiming some actual personal space.) No, I don't mean putting yourself on the step (well, you can if you want), but taking time away from your child, just for you. It's perfectly reasonable, and essential, to have some peace and quiet away from inquiring minds and chatty tongues. I have found that I don't get this unless I demand it. In less of a 'throw my-self on the ground like a two-year-old' way and more of a 'willing friend/partner/family member, do you think you could look after the kids for a few hours so I can reclaim 2 per cent of my sanity?' way. I know a few hours isn't always possible, so sometimes I've compromised and asked my three kids to entertain one another for half an hour whilst I've laid down on my bed and read a book or just relished the time not being touched or spoken to. (If you don't have other children, and your child is old enough to be left alone for a little while, CBeebies can have the same effect.) You are allowed this and you *do* deserve it.

SURVIVING TOUGH TIMES

Some days we thrive, other days we just about survive. It's all part of the colourful tapestry of being a mum and it's completely nor-mal to feel like this. Even if we *are* able to keep this in mind, the tough times – when illness hits you/your child or sleep takes a back-seat for any number of reasons, from teething to straightening out bedsheets – can be *really* tough and hit you hard. Always evaluate your life on a moment by moment basis, not a 'we did it like this yesterday so we'll do it like this again today' principle. Be flexible. Cut yourself some slack. And a slice of cake. Have a rest if you can. Don't let your thoughts become catastrophic (more on this in a bit). It's just a day, and it's going to feel so much better than this really, really soon.

GET SOME SLEEP

Even when we do get the opportunity, getting a decent night's sleep is a thing lots of us are dreadful at. If you've ever found your-self still faffing around at midnight, despite the fact your child has been asleep for several hours, you'll know what I'm talking about. GO TO BED EARLIER. The hours between 10.00 pm and 2.00 am are when our bodies renew and repair cells. We need this time to keep healthy, prevent disease and age well. Four golden hours of sleep. Do your faffing about at 2.15 am, if you must.

EAT WELL(ISH)

We can be our own worst enemies when it comes to eating. We do stuff like miss breakfast in the rush of trying to get out of the house. Or we just don't get around to lunch. Our blood sugar drops and we get HANGRY, lose concentration and our patience. So we binge on something sweet/anything that's to hand because we're suddenly starving and knackered. Realistically, it's not always going to be possible to eat well, but keeping some healthy quick snacks in the cupboard can help us make a better nutritional choice in the moment. Oatcakes. Peanut butter. Bananas. Some nuts. A piece of rye bread. A pre-boiled egg. Stuff we can grab on the go that will give us a little more sustenance and the energy to nurture others. You can only go so far on an empty tank.

RUN, FORREST, FUN

Whether you *enjoy* exercise or not isn't really the point (sorry to say that so bluntly). It's good for you and those amazing post-workout endorphins alone are totally worth the effort and enough to keep you coming back for more. They're addictive. You don't have to run a marathon or be a top athlete. A jog. A walk. A swim. Yoga. Pilates. A crazy HIIT session. *Whatever* you fancy. All have the same benefits – getting your body moving, your blood pumping and creating a stronger body and mind. Mix up your exercise to keep yourself motivated. A stronger body makes raising children so much more doable and enjoyable.

BELIEVE IN YOURSELF

Because if you don't, no one else will either. You are pretty amazing and capable of every little thing you put your marvellous mind to. True story. (You can never hear this enough, so I'll keep saying it.)

WHEN MUMS DIET...

'I'm watching what I eat.
So I'm going to miss dinner.
And just have this
bottle of prosecco,
fourteen custard creams
and a leftover
fish finger.'

ON THIS DAY

DATE: _____

Often, the only way to get some time out is to just take it.

MY NOTES
(WHAT I LOVED, FELT, WISHED, NEEDED, STRUGGLED WITH, OVERCAME)

....

....

....

....

....

....

....

....

TO DO LIST

- ☐ ....
- ☐ ....
- ☐ ....
- ☐ ....

....

....

....

- ☐ ....

THINGS TO REMEMBER
(THAT I'LL PROBABLY STILL FORGET)

....
....
....
....
....

MY SELF-CARE PLAN
(THINGS I NEED TO BE MINDFUL OF)

....
....
....
....
....

FUNNY THINGS YOU DID/SAID
(THANKS FOR MAKING ME LAUGH)

....
....
....
....
....
....
....
....
....
....
....
....

WHAT I WANT YOU TO KNOW
(YEARS FROM NOW)

....
....
....
....
....
....
....
....
....
....
....
....

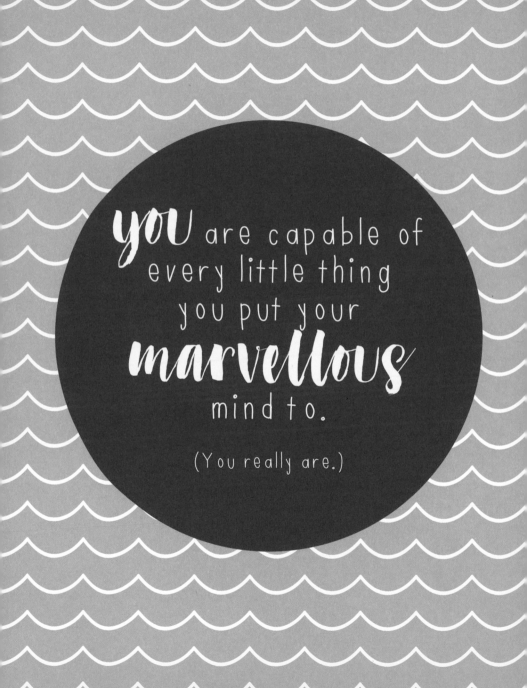

you are capable of
every little thing
you put your
marvellous
mind to.

(You really are.)

ON THIS DAY

DATE: _____

Don't be scared of exercise. MOVE your body in any way that feels good.

MY NOTES
(WHAT I LOVED, FELT, WISHED, NEEDED, STRUGGLED WITH, OVERCAME)

....

....

....

....

....

....

....

....

TO DO LIST

❏ ....

❏ ....

❏ ....

❏ ....

❏ ....

THE NOT-SO-NEW MUM'S SUPERFOOD BRUNCH

What did we do before the avocado? It's the most Instagrammed fruit, apparently. Well, I have no idea, as I probably eat it five days out of seven. Avocado is great for so many things. It's full of vitamins, including C, E and K (for osteoporosis prevention), and good fats to help you feel fuller for longer, as well as magnesium, potassium and folates, which are beneficial for pregnancy and also help lower the risk of depression. Kale is right up there with the avocado with its many powerful nutritional benefits. It's also really high in iron. The rye bread is a good carbohydrate option and the egg is full of protein and tastes blooming good. In summary? This is a brunch/lunch or anytime meal to give you a proper boost and there are so many variations you can experiment with. Substitute the egg for feta, cheddar, smoked salmon or halloumi. It all works!

CRUSHED AVOCADO ON RYE BREAD WITH KALE AND EGG

Serves one

1/2 avocado

Squeeze of lemon juice

3 handfuls of kale

Small glug of olive oil

Salt (optional)

1 egg

2 slices rye bread

Optional extras: tomatoes, baby spinach

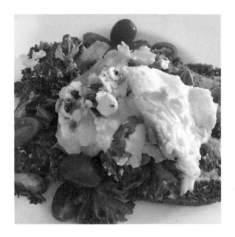

Scoop out the flesh from the avocado half and mash with the lemon juice. Stir-fry the kale in a little olive oil with a touch of salt (optional) and crack the egg into the frying pan (this will take a few minutes to cook). Meanwhile, toast the rye bread lightly, spread the avocado all over it, top with the egg and any extras and serve the kale on the side or on top. Tuck in and feel the nutrients flood your bloodstream.

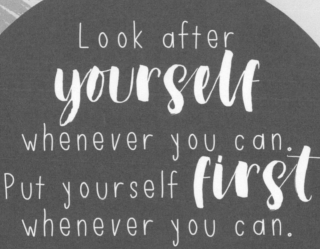

Look after **yourself** whenever you can. Put yourself **first** whenever you can.

(It will stand you in good stead.)

ON THIS DAY

DATE: _____

When you DO get the chance for sleep, SLEEP. (Don't waste it on Facebook.)

MY NOTES
(WHAT I LOVED, FELT, WISHED, NEEDED, STRUGGLED WITH, OVERCAME)

....

....

....

....

....

....

....

....

....

....

....

TO DO LIST

☐ ....

☐ ....

☐ ....

☐ ....

☐ ....

THINGS TO REMEMBER
(THAT I'LL PROBABLY STILL FORGET)

....
....
....
....
....

LIST OF EXERCISE CLASSES
(THAT I WOULD QUITE LIKE TO TRY)

....
....
....
....
....

FUNNY THINGS YOU DID/SAID
(THANKS FOR MAKING ME LAUGH)

....
....
....
....
....
....
....
....
....
....
....
....
....

WHAT I WANT YOU TO KNOW
(YEARS FROM NOW)

....
....
....
....
....
....
....
....
....
....
....
....

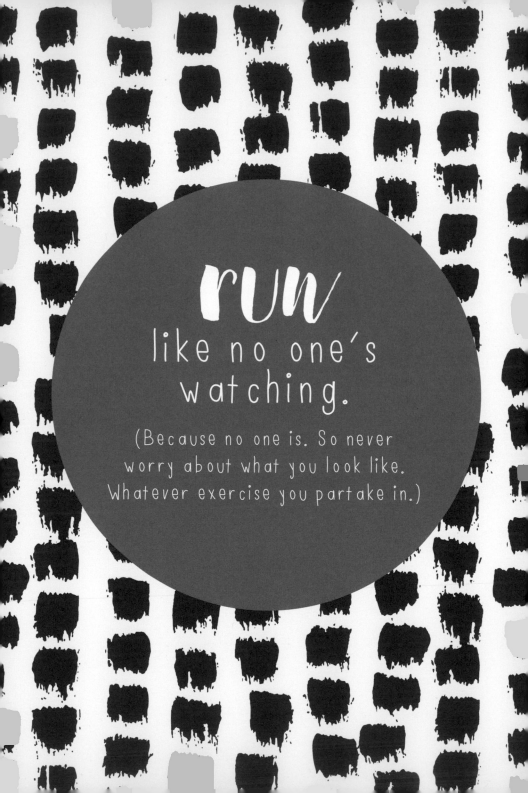

run
like no one's watching.

(Because no one is. So never
worry about what you look like.
Whatever exercise you partake in.)

ON THIS DAY

Have you drunk
enough
water today?

DATE: _____

MY NOTES
(WHAT I LOVED, FELT, WISHED, NEEDED, STRUGGLED WITH, OVERCAME)

....
....
....
....
....
....
....

TO DO LIST

- ☐ ....
- ☐ ....
....
- ☐ ....
....
- ☐ ....
....
- ☐ ....

SMALL THINGS TO LIFT YOUR MOOD

Low moods affect us all at one time or another, especially amidst the demands of motherhood. A low mood can be really debilitating and have a snowball effect on your thoughts; once it takes hold, it can be difficult to escape. But there *are* small things you can do to get yourself *happy* again. Clever, thinky, psychologist-type people always suggest lifting your mood before anything else. So here's a list of things that can help when you need to do just that.

1. Paint your nails. A great activity that allows your thoughts to switch off as you concentrate and focus on the task in hand. Plus you'll feel like you've done something for yourself, and having something bright to look at is an immediate mood lifter.

2. Slap on some lipstick. As above. A splash of colour. And it can be done regardless of budget and where you are on the baby-weight-loss scale. Amen to that.

3. Put the washing away. Yes, I know. Crazy, right? The dullest chore you've been putting off forever can actually really make a massive difference to your surroundings, and your mood. And, once you 'just do it', you realise it only takes about 5 minutes and you wonder why you've been procrastinating for so long. Plus it's hilarious to see the confused look on your child's face when they ask why all their clothes are in a drawer, because they're so used to retrieving them from piles in every room in the house.

4. De-clutter. Dealing with all the stuff that is threatening to suffocate you is so good for the soul. Recycle the junk mail that's accumulated behind the radiator and the kids' artwork that won't fit on a fridge already buckling under all the self-expression (just don't get caught binning it). Clear out old toys to donate to your local charity shop, including those annoying plastic Happy Meal or magazine figures that your child has never touched again. Put on eBay the clothes that your child has outgrown. Any sort of de-cluttering activity will make you feel truly virtuous.

5. Treat yourself. When money is tight, get yourself down to a good charity shop and pick up a new outfit for under a fiver. It's a great way to invigorate yourself, your wardrobe and do some good.

6. Tidy the garden/yard/balcony. De-weed. Sweep up leaves. Put all the toys away in a storage box. Water pots. This has totally the same effect as de-cluttering your house. And, if you get your child to help it doubles up as an activity to do together (even if it does take three times as long and you both get soaking wet).

7. Refresh your living room. When we spend a lot of time at home, our environment can start to make us feel a bit claustrophobic. We desperately crave a change of scenery. We fantasise about redecorating. Moving house. But it doesn't need to be as grand a gesture as that. Sometimes the smallest things can make the biggest difference. Get some new sofa cushions. Move the furniture around. Hang a different picture. Anything that makes your home feel 'new'.

8. Do something creative. Most of us have a creative streak, even if we don't realise it. I'm not talking about doing stuff with glitter and chalk here (most of us *don't* have that desire). But doing something creative is good for the spirit and lowers the blood pressure. Painting, writing, cooking, playing a musical instrument (badly or otherwise), doing a Bollywood dance class... set yourself free.

9. Read a book you can't put down. Reading is something we seem to do less of when we become mothers. Possibly because the constant interruptions from a small person has reduced our concentration span to 30-second intervals. Allowing yourself to get lost in a good book is pure escapism at its best. We *do* have time to read. We just often choose to look at social media instead.

10. Get mindful. Get moving. Download a mindfulness app and commit to just 10 minutes a day. Or, if you can't get out to do some uplifting exercise, get yourself on YouTube and search for a virtual Yoga or HIIT session.

11. Do less, not more. Often, when we're feeling in a bit of a funk, we need to take less action, not more. So if nothing in this list (or beyond) appeases your low mood, don't try to override it. Let it wash over you. Sometimes the relief when we allow ourselves to feel whatever it is we're feeling, without resistance, is enough to lift ourselves out of it gradually. When we're ready.

ON THIS DAY

DATE: _____

Set yourself free
every day.
Know that
you CAN.

MY NOTES
(WHAT I LOVED, FELT, WISHED, NEEDED, STRUGGLED WITH, OVERCAME)

....

....

....

....

....

....

....

....

TO DO LIST

❑ ....

❑ ....

....

❑ ....

....

❑ ....

....

❑ ....

THINGS TO REMEMBER
(THAT I'LL PROBABLY STILL FORGET)

....
....
....
....
....

STUFF THAT LIFTS MY MOOD
(THAT I CAN TAP INTO WHEN I NEED TO)

....
....
....
....
....

FUNNY THINGS YOU DID/SAID
(THANKS FOR MAKING ME LAUGH)

....
....
....
....
....
....
....
....
....
....
....
....

WHAT I WANT YOU TO KNOW
(YEARS FROM NOW)

....
....
....
....
....
....
....
....
....
....
....
....

Remember the small things
that used to make
your *heart flutter*.
And do ONE thing
that makes you feel JOY.

(Your happiness matters too.)

ON THIS DAY

DATE: _____

Reward yourself often. Praise yourself ALWAYS.

MY NOTES
(WHAT I LOVED, FELT, WISHED, NEEDED, STRUGGLED WITH, OVERCAME)

....

....

....

....

....

....

....

....

....

....

....

TO DO LIST

☐ ....

☐ ....

☐ ....

☐ ....

☐ ....

YOU HAVE A RIGHT TO BE HAPPY

WOMAN FIRST, MOTHER SECOND

I'm going to share something with you that might blow your mind, as much as it did mine when I first heard the words out loud. YOU HAVE A RIGHT TO BE HAPPY. 'Well, of course I do', you might be thinking. But, do you *really* believe this? Do you put yourself first, above others, *without* guilt? Do you think about yourself and fulfilling those desires and dreams you've not actually thought about in a while? Because it is really, really easy, once we become mothers, to become martyrs in our own lives; to give ourselves completely to our children. It's an admirable gesture, but not one that necessarily serves *us* well. We take on more and more, which only reinforces the misconception that *only* we can do everything that needs doing. We forget US and how to make ourselves happy. We forget that we even have the right to be happy. We forget that we were women long before we became mothers.

THE ROLE OF THE MOTHER IS EVOLVING

Motherhood is a funny thing. Almost overnight, we change. We're going to, that's only natural and what Mother Nature requires of us in order to nurture our young. But we take it too far in an age that demands we be ALL things to ALL men (women, children and anyone else who asks). We constantly judge ourselves as mothers, partners, friends and workers. We allow ourselves to feel judged (even when no one is actually judging us) and we live under the influence of opinions, outdated traditions and our own fear and assumption that we're just not good enough. We put our happiness to the bottom of that washing pile, which refuses to go down, no matter how often we do it. We feel distanced, at times, from our own identity and occasionally (or frequently) doubt that we have the right to be happy, unless that happiness directly involves our children's. We foolishly don't recognise that if we are happy then our children are happy, *by default*, because that's how happiness works. It spreads quicker than an outbreak of chicken pox in a nursery (and is thankfully far less itchy).

JUST BE HAPPY

We do have a choice and that is simply to accept our desire and right to be happy and to go about fulfilling it with purpose and conviction. Without question. It's our *choice* if, instead, we see our roles as mothers as sacrificial and expect our children to make us happy. That's the burden right there, isn't it? That we perceive we've given everything up for them, so the least they can do is behave, eat their carrots and make our effort worthwhile. Yet, who is possibly going to win in a relationship that swings on such a paralysing and inevitably disappointing pendulum of responsibility and guilt? Surely it's far better to be kinder to ourselves, raise our children as the temporary guardians/teachers we are supposed to be, and show them the very definition of happiness and self-esteem by always valuing ourselves, rather than resenting every painful second?

IT'S NOT OUR ROLE TO MAKE EVERYTHING RIGHT

We do not own our children. We do not own their choices. We do not own their futures. It has taken me a while to realise this and think about what this means. In short, it means that it is NOT our role to make everything right in our child's world when things fall apart. It's our role to talk to them, listen to them, guide them without suffocating them (and ourselves) and highlight their strengths when they can't see them for themselves. THIS is particularly important, because if you've ever had someone in your corner, who truly and consistently believes in you, even when you mess up, you'll know what a powerful incentive it is to keep going, with pride. Acknowledging this idea – that you aren't ultimately responsible for your child's happiness – suddenly dissolves a lot of the stress and responsibility you feel as a parent. It's more intuitive and more interactive than simply reacting to what they do with reward or punishment. It's less about *telling* them and more about helping them *learn* that they are the stars of their own lives and only they can write the plot. If they can nurture this kind of self-belief early on, which all kids are born with – you only have to look at the ego of a young child to see it – there isn't going to be anything they can't handle.

A GOOD MUM IS YOU

Most mothers fall into the trap of questioning how good they are at this motherhood lark. Of comparing themselves. We feel a huge sense of achievement whenever we perceive ourselves to be 'good mums' – we've laid their clothes out the night before, played/read with them and cooked a meal from scratch. When we haven't come up with the goods because we're short of time and it's been Netflix and a beige banquet from the freezer instead, we label ourselves 'bad mums'. Why? We've still loved them the same. We've still fed, nurtured and taken care of them. Who says we, as women, don't count? Who says our own personal vision of the mother *we* are comfortable being, doesn't count? Each. To. Their. Own. Always. So, whenever you find yourself asking, 'Would a good mum do this?' as you open that bottle of wine with a friend, stick on another film in your TV marathon, or dust off yesterday's tights, the answer is most definitely, always YES. A good mum does whatever it is *she* feels comfortable doing. At that point in time. A good mum puts herself first, when she deems that it feels right and pleasurable to do so. A good mum realises that she has the right to be happy and that she is a better caregiver when she is. A good mum is YOU.

You were a *woman* before you were a mother. *nurture* her often. You can't be a 'good' mother without her.

(She's super important.)

ON THIS DAY

DATE: _____

What if we teach our children, rather than tell them?

MY NOTES
(WHAT I LOVED, FELT, WISHED, NEEDED, STRUGGLED WITH, OVERCAME)

....

....

....

....

....

....

....

....

TO DO LIST

☐ ....

☐ ....

☐ ....

☐ ....

☐ ....

THINGS TO REMEMBER
(THAT I'LL PROBABLY STILL FORGET)

....

....

....

....

....

WAYS I CAN PUT ME FIRST
(BECAUSE I HAVE A RIGHT TO BE HAPPY)

....

....

....

....

....

FUNNY THINGS YOU DID/SAID
(THANKS FOR MAKING ME LAUGH)

....

....

....

....

....

....

....

....

....

....

....

....

....

WHAT I WANT YOU TO KNOW
(YEARS FROM NOW)

....

....

....

....

....

....

....

....

....

....

....

....

....

A good mum is
you.

(In whatever shape, form or mood
you find yourself in today.)

ON THIS DAY

DATE: _____

You always
have the right
to be happy.

MY NOTES
(WHAT I LOVED, FELT, WISHED, NEEDED, STRUGGLED WITH, OVERCAME)

....

....

....

....

....

....

....

....

....

....

....

TO DO LIST

☐ ....

☐ ....

☐ ....

☐ ....

☐ ....

10 ACTIVITIES YOU CAN DO IN THE EVENING

Sometimes, after a day with kids, you want to do something *other* than watch TV/drink wine. No? You don't? Ok then, as you were, just whizz pass this page, there's never any judgement here. If, on the other hand, you *are* feeling in need of a little something else, to make you feel alive and a little invigorated, here's a list of things you can do in the evening *without* having to leave the house and pay an overpriced babysitter. In no particular order...

1. Have a bath. Sometimes, after a hectic bathtime/bedtime with a small person, the evening bath we might have promised ourselves hours, days, or even months before just doesn't happen. It feels like too much effort. But the healing powers of a warm bath are not to be underestimated. So hide all the plastic toys, light a candle, pour in some bath oil with a relaxing fragrance and lie back. Your body and mind will thank you.

2. Have a pamper evening for one. This is a step on from just having a bath. Do the whole shebang. Face mask. Hair mask. Exfoliate. Shave your legs. Scrub your feet. Moisturise. Paint your nails. Basically all the things you last did in a parallel life a long, long time ago. You can even finish it off with that mindfulness app or YouTube yoga session I mentioned earlier. Then give yourself that early night you've been promising yourself. No TV, no phones, no stimulants. You'll feel regenerated.

3. Create a picture wall. The digital age has made printing actual photos and putting them in frames a distant memory. But all these beautiful photos you take are no good sitting on a Cloud somewhere. So spend an evening downloading the pictures from your phone, picking your favourites and getting them printed. Order some picture frames then spend another evening hanging them. Picture walls can be wonderfully eclectic, with a mish-mash of frames and sizes, so you can keep adding to it, as and when you wish.

4. Start a memory box. Memories don't have to be in chronological order in scrapbooks (phew). In years to come, rifling through a wooden box jam-packed full of all your memories – from your own childhood through to adulthood and motherhood – is such a lovely way to spend an afternoon. So start now and throw in anything and everything that means something to you.

5. Breathe. When did you last breathe? I mean, properly breathe, not the quick, sharp breaths you fit in in between all the rushing. Our poor-quality breathing has so much to do with all the tension and anxiety we carry in our bodies. So take some time out to *just breathe*. Sit down, breathe in for 3 seconds and out for 5 seconds. Try to extend the length of the out breath a little more each time until you are breathing out for 10 seconds or more. Do this for 10 minutes and see how differently you feel at the end. In general, it's worth teaching yourself to be more aware of your breathing as you go about your day, taking deep in-breaths and expelling all the stale air when you have the chance..

6 Try a new recipe, Russian roulette-style. Invigorate your diet with a new recipe. Look in the fridge/cupboard, pick a few key ingredients, google the combination and see what recipes it comes up with. Then make it and eat it.

7. Have sex. If this suggestion fills you with dread or you can't remember when you last did it, it's probably been too long. We all know that intimacy is a crucial part of connecting in a relationship (if you're in one), especially once kids come along. It's also a great source of releasing tension. (Or you can just do a bit more breathing.)

8. Call a friend. They might a) not answer, or b) pick up immediately and ask, 'WHAT'S HAPPENED? IS EVERYTHING OK?' at the pure shock of someone actually calling rather than texting. We often say we don't have time to catch up with people. The truth is we just use the time to do something else instead. Put aside all the to-dos and call that person you've been wanting to speak to for ages. And drink a cup of reassuring and calming chamomile tea whilst you do.

9. Lay on your bed and listen to music. A song or piece of music has the power to transport you to another place. We usually have it on as 'noise' in the background, playing in the kitchen or the car, with kids' voices in the foreground. Dedicate some time to really listening and enjoying it. You'll probably be asleep in seconds.

10. Make a mood board for your future. This is such a brilliant way to spend an evening. Invite some friends over to really make the most of it. Get all your old magazines, a large piece of card (A3 or bigger), some scissors and glue. Divide the card into the following eight sections: Wealth/Travel (top left), Love (top right), Gratitude (below Love), Friendship (bottom right), Career (bottom middle), Knowledge/Self Development (bottom left), Family (above Knowledge/Self Development) and You (centre). Pick pictures that speak to you, that say something about the direction you want to go in each of these areas, even if you don't immediately understand how or why they appeal. Cut them out and stick them down. If you're doing it with friends and you each feel comfortable, you can share a little about what you've done at the end. Keep your mood board to hand, visualise your desires and watch them come true. It really works and it's something that people pay life coaches hundreds of pounds to help them with, but it is something you can easily do with a little of your own intuition and passion.

Feeling *passion* for something other than your child is really, really good for your *soul.*

(Let's do more of that, then.)

ON THIS DAY

DATE: _____

Have a bath at 3.00pm in the afternoon because your child's fallen asleep. Why not?

MY NOTES
(WHAT I LOVED, FELT, WISHED, NEEDED, STRUGGLED WITH, OVERCAME)

....

....

....

....

....

....

....

....

TO DO LIST

☐ ....

☐ ....

☐ ....

☐ ....

☐ ....

THINGS TO REMEMBER
(THAT I'LL PROBABLY STILL FORGET)

....
....
....
....
....

MY PERFECT EVENING
(THIS IS WHAT IT LOOKS LIKE)

....
....
....
....
....

FUNNY THINGS YOU DID/SAID
(THANKS FOR MAKING ME LAUGH)

....
....
....
....
....
....
....
....
....
....
....
....
....

WHAT I WANT YOU TO KNOW
(YEARS FROM NOW)

....
....
....
....
....
....
....
....
....
....
....
....
....

Take a moment to think how you want your *future* to look.

(Then picture it when days feel long.)

ON THIS DAY

DATE: _____

When did you last really enjoy your dinner? Make it an occasion for a change.

MY NOTES
(WHAT I LOVED, FELT, WISHED, NEEDED, STRUGGLED WITH, OVERCAME)

....

....

....

....

....

....

....

....

....

....

....

TO DO LIST

❑ ....

❑ ....

❑ ....

❑ ....

❑ ....

TO WORK OR NOT TO WORK?

THERE'S NO PERFECT SCENARIO

The life of a working mum is never an easy one. Then again, nor is the life of a stay-at-home mum. I think it is fair to say that there is no perfect scenario that suits all, just the one that works *best* for you and your family. (And you might not even like that one, some days.)

STAYING AT HOME

For some mums, 'staying at home' to look after their child(ren) is what they always planned or hoped to do. For others, it is a complete surprise as they discover motherhood fulfils them in a way they hadn't expected. They are mostly completely content (aside from the tough days we all have). Yet, as women strive ever more for equality and their share of opportunities, choosing to stay at home isn't understood by everyone in a society that perhaps doesn't always regard motherhood as the incredibly important role that it is. We are more likely to talk about motherhood not being enough than how amazing it is to have the privilege of shaping these small minds every day. It can leave mums, for whom motherhood is more than enough, justifying their decision or 'what they do all day' (anyone who asks a mum *this* has clearly never been one). If you want to stay at home with your kids, and are able to do it financially, then there is no other place you should be.

JUGGLING WORK AND MOTHERHOOD

Mums go back to work for a host of different reasons. Financial reasons. Career. Sanity. If you went back to work after your maternity leave, you'll already know the benefits and challenges that this presents. The tight schedule, commuting, nursery runs, your child being ill, childminders and nannies taking sick days, all on top of trying to do an actual job that satisfies your employer. There are days where you wonder, 'Is this *really* worth it?' as you hand over the best part of your salary to your childcare provider. Of course, the goal is a much longer-term one because there will come a time, actually not that far away, when your child will be in school and your salary will be your own again (sort of). Juggling work and motherhood is no small feat – some days it is EPIC – and you should remember how amazing you are for balancing all of this, every single day. Especially when the fridge is empty, the washing basket is overflowing and the bin is drawing attention to itself with a smell that can only be described as putrid. Or when you're late (again), shouting at everyone at the same time as calling your local railway station to ask if they'd mind holding the train. All while *Snow White* (aka your three-year-old) finishes accessorising. Because it doesn't matter *how* late you are: when you're three, there's *always* time to worry about which necklace or superhero mask you are going to wear. So when you're on the verge of that meltdown and feeling overwhelmed by it all, STEP BACK. Don't focus on what you *aren't* managing to do but look at what you're achieving instead. EPIC, that's you. Every single day.

MISSING WORK (AND MAYBE GOING BACK)

You possibly didn't ever think you'd see these two words side by side. Before you became a mother, maybe this was the DREAM. Giving it all up, raising your child(ren) and baking a pie. Then you woke up, realised you aren't a 1950s housewife and wondered why The Motherhood Dream isn't quite as fulfilling as you'd anticipated. PERFECTLY NORMAL. You find yourself missing work, your colleagues, hot coffee, having a wee on your own and time to be you. It's natural to sometimes wish for whatever situation isn't your own. Some days, the grass isn't just greener on the other side, it's a vibrant shade of neon. If you're thinking about going back to work after more than a year out, the thought can be pretty terrifying. You might have lost some confidence in yourself and your abilities. Well, STOP. RIGHT. THERE. Mothers are the most resourceful and efficient beings on the planet (apart from when we're forgetful, late, or don't turn up at all). We're Queens of Multi-Tasking and getting stuff done. That boss you used to find tricky? They're nothing in comparison to a threenager who can negotiate so hard they should work for the FBI. Being a working mum takes determination, organisation and commitment (so does being a stay-at-home mum). You have this in abundance. So if you're thinking of returning to work, be tenacious about it. Show your potential employer what an asset you'd be. Because you are. If, on the other hand, you're having a lie down after reading this, then perhaps it's not quite the right time for you. Yet. That's ok. Be confident in your choice to be with your child(ren), especially when the tough days hit and make you question everything. For now, you just need a temporary escape plan that you can enact for a few moments at home: close the toilet door (by which I mean barricade it shut) and breathe.

WHEN YOU BOTH WORK

Balancing two careers within a family can be really demanding. There's less flexibility for you both and you can find yourself at loggerheads when a child is sick and needs one of you to leave work. So often, this responsibility still falls to the mother; a combination of society's expectations and possibly the fact that you haven't sat down together and talked about how curveballs like this will be dealt with. Resentment can build quickly in a relationship where both parents work, if one perceives or infers that their job is more important or more valuable because they earn more. Making a flexible plan can help you figure out how you will share the nursery runs/sick days so that both partners feel equal and appreciated.

WHEN YOU'RE THE BREADWINNER

If you're the breadwinner and your partner is staying at home to look after your child, you may find yourself feeling a bit out of your depth; that you're not in the loop. When did your child start doing that? Did you even notice? How come all those other mums are using *exactly* the same snacks? When did all those other parents get to be such good friends? I remember this feeling well when I was working almost full-time and I had to get to work, which basically meant I never saw any other parents. Ever. I imagined they were all drinking coffee, having a marvellous time and talking about how much they loved nursery rhymes and those special snacks. Since becoming freelance, and being able to hang out with other mums and dads as much as I like and also be at the school gates EVERY SINGLE DAY (which can be painful enough in itself), I can assure you nothing *that* exciting happens. No one's partying like it's 1999. No one is BFFs with anyone else. Everyone's just doing the best they can. Don't put pressure on yourself. Don't allow yourself to feel bad. You're doing what you need to do for your family and that's just marvellous. Focus on *that*.

STARTING UP YOUR OWN BUSINESS

I think motherhood brings out a creative side in us. It certainly brings out a desire to find that elusive work-life-motherhood balance. It's why there are so many inspirational and determined women setting up their own businesses post-baby and making such a success of them – because of that wonderful resourcefulness and efficiency we each possess. It can be scary starting up something on your own, but if you have an idea that makes so much sense to you that you can't *not* believe in it, that compels you to get on with it without even talking it through with the world, then what are you waiting for? There is a theory that ideas belong to individuals and are given to us. If we don't pursue them, they're given to someone else. Isn't it magical to think that the idea simmering away inside of you is meant for you, first and foremost?

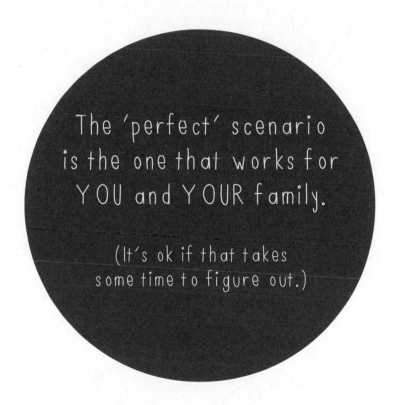

The 'perfect' scenario
is the one that works for
YOU and YOUR family.

(It's ok if that takes
some time to figure out.)

ON THIS DAY

DATE: _____

Juggling work and motherhood is totally enough. Take easy options wherever you can.

MY NOTES
(WHAT I LOVED, FELT, WISHED, NEEDED, STRUGGLED WITH, OVERCAME)

....

....

....

....

....

....

....

TO DO LIST

.... ☐ ....

.... ☐ ....

.... ☐ ....

.... ☐ ....

.... ☐ ....

THINGS TO REMEMBER
(THAT I'LL PROBABLY STILL FORGET)

....
....
....
....
....

MY HOPES AND DREAMS
(WHAT I'D LIKE FOR THE FUTURE)

....
....
....
....
....

FUNNY THINGS YOU DID/SAID
(THANKS FOR MAKING ME LAUGH)

....
....
....
....
....
....
....
....
....
....
....
....

WHAT I WANT YOU TO KNOW
(YEARS FROM NOW)

....
....
....
....
....
....
....
....
....
....
....
....

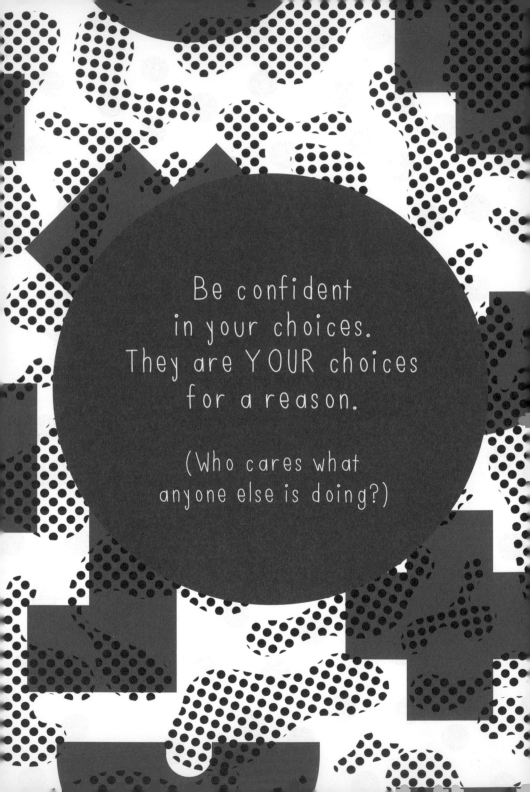

Be confident
in your choices.
They are YOUR choices
for a reason.

(Who cares what
anyone else is doing?)

ON THIS DAY

You should
be really proud of
all you hold down.
(It's a lot.)

DATE: _____

MY NOTES
(WHAT I LOVED, FELT, WISHED, NEEDED, STRUGGLED WITH, OVERCAME)

....

....

....

....

....

....

....

....

....

....

....

TO DO LIST

❏ ....

❏ ....

❏ ....

❏ ....

❏ ....

STARTING CHILDCARE AND TRUSTING OTHERS

Your child starting nursery, preschool or spending time with a nanny or childminder is a major milestone. If you went back to work after maternity leave, you'll remember this and also how stressful the process can be. If your child's yet to start, you'll want to be as prepared as you can be so you can avoid having a nervous breakdown in the process. Here are a few pointers from someone who's done it three times (me!) and been at nursery for approximately 79 years. Ha ha.

LOOKING FOR 'THE ONE'

Find a nursery or childminder you love. Like REALLY love. As in, you'd happily marry them and live happily ever after. This is going to help you feel a million times better when it comes to leaving your child. If you're coming back from a nursery wondering if one of the nursery workers was stoned (ahem), it's probably time to keep looking. I visited ten nurseries before I found The One. And I just knew the moment I stepped through the door of The Nursery on the Green. It felt like home. In fact, I loved it so much that some days I wished I could stay there, instead of going off to work. I've only just left, after 8 years and three kids, and I owe them so much for helping me raise three confident children. Good nurseries fill up quickly, so you'll need to get your name down WAY in advance of when you'd like to start. And don't forget, when your child hits 3 years, you're likely to be eligible for some free hours each week. Hurrah!

SETTLING THEM (AND YOU)

Most childcare providers will give you a period of time in which to settle your child. Each one does this slightly differently, but it will go something like this. You'll go together the first time for an hour, then the next day you will stay with them for, say, half an hour and leave them for another half hour. The third day you'll leave them for a bit longer, if not for the whole day/session. Parting company isn't always easy, for either of you. Some kids cry whilst others don't give a hoot. They're all different. I'm not sure if the criers do it to a) make us feel guilty; b) because they love us so darn much; or c) because they're hungry/tired/not happy with their sock choice that morning. It's beyond excruciating for the parent, but do NOT hang around, no matter how great the temptation. It prolongs the agony for you and for them. You can pretty much guarantee that the moment you've closed the door behind you, sobbing, they're totally over it. My third was at nursery for a year before he stopped crying when I left him (sorry). I was obviously very jaded by this point, so I just smiled, patted him on the head and RAN. In other words? You'll get used to it too. I promise.

THE FIRST FULL DAY/SESSION

It is SO easy to spend their first full day thinking about them, even if you're at work in the midst of a really important meeting. Are they ok? Have they eaten? Did they nap? Resist the urge to phone every 5 minutes and keep busy instead. Then make a call halfway into their session and check in on them.

MISSING MILESTONES

One of the things lots of parents worry about is missing those oh so important milestones. What if your child starts walking and you miss those first steps or they learn to hold a pen properly and you didn't witness it? Well, there is a code amongst most nurseries, nannies and childminders that they'll keep this to themselves and let you experience the joy for yourself. Nice, eh?

BE FLEXIBLE

Your childcare will likely do things differently to you. Whilst they will do their best to adhere to any particular routine you follow, they have other children to take into consideration and you may need to be willing to compromise. I remember my first child starting nursery. I told them she was a 'Gina Ford' baby and she had to nap at an exact time in complete darkness and silence. There was NO WAY they could replicate this in a busy nursery environment. Needless to say, on the first day they called me to say she had been very unsettled but it was ok because they had eventually got her to sleep by rocking her in a buggy. WHAT?! This is supposedly one of the biggest sins in the 'routine baby' book and I think I actually believed the world would end if I ever allowed it to happen. So of course I completely FREAKED out. Weeks later, when my daughter had adjusted, she slept there happily in a cot and, guess what, the world was still spinning. Eight years on, as a now somewhat slack mum of three who usually forgets parents' evening (and everything else), me and my nursery laughed about this. A LOT.

GIVE THEM YOUR TRUST

The childcare you've chosen deserves to have your trust; the relationship doesn't work unless they do. Always raise anything that's niggled you, preferably when you're calm enough to talk it through sensibly. Because, sometimes, the strength of our emotions towards our children can cloud our judgement. Accept that things will not be perfect ALL of the time. Nothing and no one ever is. You can always find fault with something, if you look hard enough, and sometimes other parents may try to rile you or sow seeds of doubt by discussing their personal gripes with you (this also happens once you get to school). I've never found this helps anyone; it's unfair, poisonous and usually nothing to do with your own, or your child's, experience. Remember why YOU picked your childcare and so long as you're happy, all is well.

FEEL GOOD ABOUT IT

Guilt is a mother's prerogative, we already know that. But don't give in to it and continually analyse whether you're doing the right thing leaving your child, especially if you're not working and using the childcare for YOU time. You do not have to justify your reasons to anyone else, or even yourself. Nurseries, nannies and childminders provide amazing, diverse environments for your child. They also do tons of wild stuff you'd *never* do at home, like sensory play with sand indoors (I'm coming out in hives just thinking about that).

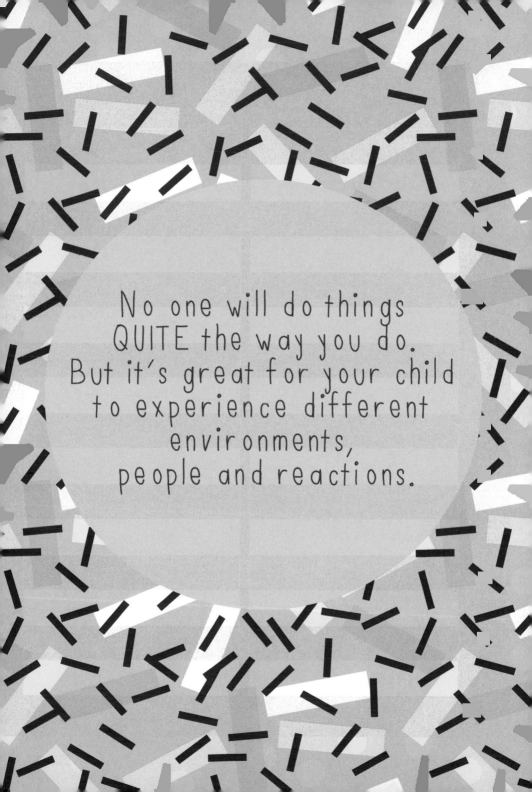

No one will do things
QUITE the way you do.
But it's great for your child
to experience different
environments,
people and reactions.

ON THIS DAY

DATE: _____

Try to get a recommendation for childcare if you can.

MY NOTES
(WHAT I LOVED, FELT, WISHED, NEEDED, STRUGGLED WITH, OVERCAME)

....

....

....

....

....

....

....

....

....

....

....

TO DO LIST

☐ ....

☐ ....

☐ ....

☐ ....

☐ ....

THINGS TO REMEMBER
(THAT I'LL PROBABLY STILL FORGET)

....
....
....
....
....

NURSERIES AND NANNIES
(THAT I WOULD LIKE TO CHECK OUT)

....
....
....
....
....

FUNNY THINGS YOU DID/SAID
(THANKS FOR MAKING ME LAUGH)

....
....
....
....
....
....
....
....
....
....
....
....
....

WHAT I WANT YOU TO KNOW
(YEARS FROM NOW)

....
....
....
....
....
....
....
....
....
....
....
....
....

Remember
absence makes
the heart grow
fonder.
Enjoy every reunion
and make your time
together count.

ON THIS DAY

DATE:

Never get drawn into nursery or childcare politics.

MY NOTES
(WHAT I LOVED, FELT, WISHED, NEEDED, STRUGGLED WITH, OVERCAME)

....
....
....
....
....
....
....

....

....

....

....

TO DO LIST

☐ ....

☐ ....

☐ ....

☐ ....

☐ ....

PLEASE GO AWAY, ANXIETY (THANK YOU)

WHEN ANXIETY HITS

If you're reading this as an anxiety sufferer, I want to give you a big hug and tell you that your inner strength knows no bounds. YOU ARE A WARRIOR. Anxiety is a miserable and debilitating state of being; it warps your rational thought, it cripples your confidence and it makes you feel so unwell that you doubt everything you thought you knew. It strikes without warning and it affects the way you live your life and the decisions you take. If you've recently started suffering from anxiety, please know that you are *not* alone. There isn't a mum in the world who hasn't felt anxious at some point. About life. About work. About her health. About dying and leaving her kids and her other half not knowing that a potato isn't actually 'one of your five a day'. For so many mums, these thoughts are a daily soundtrack in their lives. YOU ARE NOT ALONE.

DEALING WITH ANXIETY

Our natural reaction to anxiety is to feel fear, or FEAR: False Evidence Appearing Real. Which is basically what anxiety is: something that probably isn't going to happen, except in our minds. The fear brings on all those unpleasant physical symptoms that scare us so much: the dizziness; the nausea; the difficulty breathing – or that general state of feeling unwell, which further convinces us that something must be *really* wrong. On a primitive level, this is the fight or flight response kicking in, but rarely are we in a situation where we are actually in immediate danger. So, in our modern lives, where we aren't running around in loin cloths being chased by lions, we have to learn how to manage this; to be able to figure out what's real and what's not. The thing about anxious thoughts is that they always pass – experience teaches us this much because we survived the previous attack – usually once you've accepted them and allowed your brain to rationalise them, rather than fighting against them (which can instead increase the fear and fight or flight response). Thankfully, health anxiety, for example, is particularly receptive to rationale. That headache you've

306

got; the dizziness; the exhaustion: what if it's something serious? Or, more likely, what if it's because you're dehydrated, tired and stretched, you forgot to eat (again) and you're just not looking after yourself as well as you should be. The moment that you build that very rational list of reasons in your mind, the relief washes over you and the physical symptoms you're feeling start to fade. Changing your focus is also incredibly effective. So, if you're suddenly anxious about the nursery run, that email you didn't send or whatever it is, instead of remembering how you felt *last* time, you think about something completely different. Something sensory, such as how your coat/scarf/bag feels – examine every fibre. Finally, paying attention to your breathing always works. Take 10 minutes or so to breathe. ACTUALLY BREATHE. Not the shallow, poor quality breathing we so often jam in amidst all the rushing. But proper breathing that fills every bit of your lungs. Three seconds in and 5 seconds out, extending your breath a little each time until you settle on a length that feels right for you in that moment. It's the simplest, most immediate thing we can do for ourselves in anxious times.

LIVING WITH ANXIETY

Even when you've recovered, even when you are well, even when you are vigilant about maintaining your mental well-being (which isn't always easy as a time-pressured, often sleep-deprived mum), the reality is that once you've suffered from anxiety (or depression), unfortunately you are more likely to suffer from it again. Medication, CBT and therapy absolutely helps, but it can sometimes feel like it's failing you in the midst of an anxiety attack or when you feel so low you can't face getting out of bed. Persevere and also learn to be more accepting of yourself. Treat an anxious or low day as just that. One day. Go with it rather than resist or fear it. Realise that, in many ways, you are who you are *because* of your anxiety, not despite it. Once you start to emerge from the fog again, you can regain your perspective on who you are and who you want to be. And you know that you can handle *anything* because you've reached rock bottom before and made your way back up. You will never stop doing this. You will always go on.

COPING WITH RELAPSES

If you ever feel like you're relapsing, get to work on identifying your triggers immediately, before it takes hold and becomes so much harder to see. A change in circumstances. Illness. Medication. Diet (sugar can aggravate mood and hormone levels). Contraception. Your hormonal cycle (try a 'monthly cycle' app to track any patterns – pre-ovulation can be tricky for some). Caffeine. Alcohol. Sleep patterns. All of these factors (and more) are critical when you're predisposed to mental health issues. Then, decide to make the effort to take one day at a time, and to make that day pleasurable in some small way, whether that's going for a walk in the fresh air, getting a nice drink or seeing a friend. Using a mindfulness app, especially one with an 'anxiety' programme, for 10 minutes every day really helps. We have the power to make sure that every moment, every 'now', is worth concentrating on in some small way. And we're doing ourselves good when we do this because those pleasurable moments lift the mood, increase the serotonin and make it a little bit harder for those anxious thoughts to seep in. If you aren't able to do this – and sometimes it may not be enough – speak to your doctor or a counsellor. Just because you had help once, it doesn't mean you won't need it again. Relapses are common and nothing to be ashamed of.

PND DOESN'T JUST HAPPEN TO NEW MUMS

There is a misconception that you can only have post-natal depression if you're a new mum with a small baby in tow. The term 'post-natal' really just refers to *when* it occurs – after having a baby. Beyond that, it's depression and it can happen to any mum, at any time, for any reason (or even none at all), just like it can to anyone else. Sadly, there are a lot of 'new mums' who remain undiagnosed and who, 2, 3 or 6 years into motherhood, are still feeling out of sorts or really unwell and just become so used to it that they no longer question it. In this respect, it is totally possible to have PND as a 'Not-So-New mum', because it never went away in the first place. If you have any of these persistent symptoms – frequent tearfulness, anxiety, health anxiety, panic attacks, insomnia, lethargy, a sense of doom, hopelessness or being unable to cope and/or physical symptoms such as muscle aches, headaches, dizziness – it might be time to talk to a friend, a GP or anyone you trust. You don't have to feel like this. You don't ever have to suffer.

TRY NOT TO DWELL ON
anxious thoughts.
TODAY IS A DAY
WHERE YOU CAN DO
anything.

(Even if it doesn't feel like it.)

ON THIS DAY

DATE: _____

Every morning, say aloud what you are grateful for.

MY NOTES
(WHAT I LOVED, FELT, WISHED, NEEDED, STRUGGLED WITH, OVERCAME)

....

....

....

....

....

....

....

....

....

....

....

TO DO LIST

☐ ....

☐ ....

☐ ....

☐ ....

☐ ....

THINGS TO REMEMBER
(THAT I'LL PROBABLY STILL FORGET)

....
....
....
....
....

MY ANXIETY TRIGGERS
(SO I CAN KEEP A LOOK OUT)

....
....
....
....
....

FUNNY THINGS YOU DID/SAID
(THANKS FOR MAKING ME LAUGH)

....
....
....
....
....
....
....
....
....
....
....
....
....

WHAT I WANT YOU TO KNOW
(YEARS FROM NOW)

....
....
....
....
....
....
....
....
....
....
....
....
....

Breathe.
Three seconds in.
Five seconds out.
Repeat.
10 times.
Feel calmer.

ON THIS DAY

DATE: _____

Frame your day with a positive goal.

MY NOTES
(WHAT I LOVED, FELT, WISHED, NEEDED, STRUGGLED WITH, OVERCAME)

....

....

....

....

....

....

....

....

....

....

....

TO DO LIST

❏ ....

❏ ....

❏ ....

❏ ....

❏ ....

HORMONES, PMT AND SMALL KIDS WHO WANT TO TOUCH YOU

Ah. The joys of the monthly cycle. The joys of being a woman. The joys of being a mother with the most GOD ALMIGHTY PMT you've ever had, whilst juggling small kids who just want to touch you constantly. It is perfectly fine not to want to have *anyone* around you when PMT strikes (and that includes your child). Here's a list of other things that are also perfectly fine. Just in case you were wondering. Ahem.

1. Not explaining stuff. Nope. You're not doing it. You're not answering any questions which start with 'why'. The explaining portion of this part of motherhood is temporarily suspended.

2. Not negotiating stuff. Your child tries to negotiate any number of things with you, from dinner choices to bathtime as you resist the urge to scream, 'ARE YOU EFFING KIDDING ME!' while staring wildly back. Strangely, your usually non-compliant threenager who does a *really* good job of playing the innocent fool most of the time, now seems to know *exactly* what you're asking. Funny, that.

3. Not moving from the sofa. Even if you wanted to move, you couldn't. But you don't want to, so there's nothing more to say.

4. Baking a whole chocolate cake to eat yourself in one sitting. You've eaten everything else remotely chocolatey in the house (including the out-of-date sprinkles). And you cannot bear the thought of leaving the house in order to get more. So you do the next best thing: you bake an entire chocolate cake, ice it and eat it. In one go. You, who didn't have the energy to get off the sofa earlier to pick up a piece of Lego for your angry-not-as-angry-as-you toddler. (The recipe for your very own PMT chocolate feast is on page 316.)

5. Refusing to discuss sanitary protection with a three-year-old.
'What's that string hanging down, Mummy?' This is never going to
end well. One question will lead to another and anyway, if there was
ONE MILLISECOND OF YOUR LIFE where you'd like to use the toilet
in peace, this one is it.

6. Imposing a touching ban. Being touched on your period by a
really small intrusive person with no awareness of the notion of personal space *actually physically* hurts. So you hide under the kitchen
table with your massive chocolate cake and sob in between shovel-
ling down large mouthfuls.

7. Throwing all the plastic tat away, whilst ranting loudly. Standing
on a piece of Lego (that piece you couldn't be bothered to pick
up earlier, oh the irony), sends you into intervals of blind rage and
tears. But you get your own back by stomping angrily around the
room, bin-bagging anything plastic in your path, whilst your child
looks on in a curious, 'Oops, Mummy's lost the plot' kind of way.

8. Sending angry texts to your partner at work. Who doesn't
enjoy an angry text? So when you get the 'I'm going to be a bit late
tonight' message, you reply with a bunch of expletives that all start
with C. And 'Chocolate' isn't one of them.

'PMT MY KIDS ARE IRRITATING ME' CHOCOLATE CAKE

Best eaten in one go, in any room that has a lock on the door or where small people can't find you.

FOR THE SPONGE
3 eggs
200g butter
200g caster sugar
150g self-raising flour
50g cocoa powder

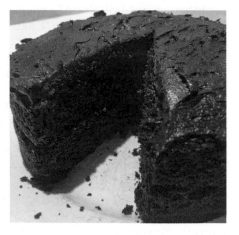

Set the oven to 180°C/Gas Mark 4. Put all the ingredients in a food processor together and mix until blended. I've also made this in a saucepan with a hand-held whisk (don't ask). Divide into two 20cm (8 inch) cake tins and bake for about 18 minutes (if you're using larger tins, bake for slightly less time). If you don't have greaseproof paper (I never do), butter the cake tins and just tip the sponges out onto plates or a wire rack as soon as they come out of the oven.

FOR THE ICING
100g icing sugar
50g soft butter
25g cocoa powder
3 tablespoons milk
4 squares dark/milk chocolate

SERVES ONE
(OR EIGHT PEOPLE WITHOUT PMT)

Mix the icing sugar, butter and cocoa together. Add the milk and mix again. Melt the chocolate in a heatproof bowl set over a pan of simmering water with the base of the bowl not touching the water. Remove and leave to cool then pour into the icing mixture. Spread half on one of the sponges, sandwich the two sponges together and spread the rest of the icing over the top. If you don't have all of these ingredients, lashings of jam will work well in the middle.

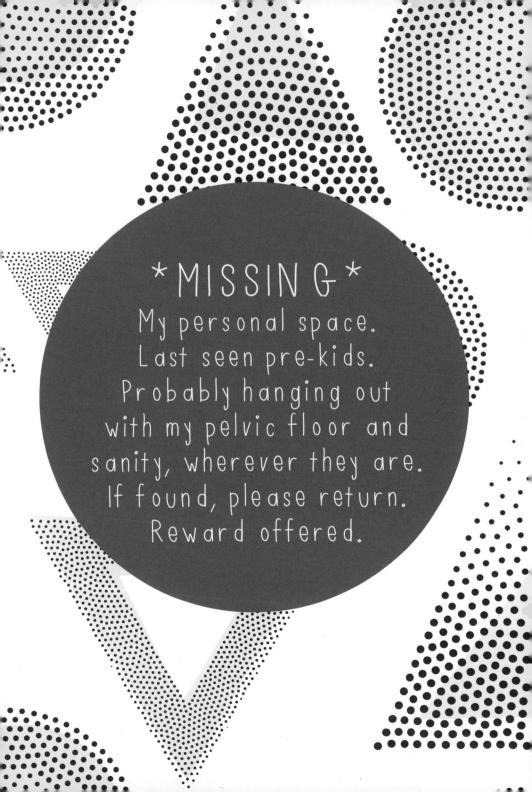

ON THIS DAY

DATE: _____

When you need some physical space, take 5 minutes out. It will do wonders.

MY NOTES
(WHAT I LOVED, FELT, WISHED, NEEDED, STRUGGLED WITH, OVERCAME)

....

....

....

....

....

....

....

....

....

....

....

....

TO DO LIST

❑ ....

❑ ....

❑ ....

❑ ....

❑ ....

THINGS TO REMEMBER
(THAT I'LL PROBABLY STILL FORGET)

....
....
....
....
....

STUFF I'M GRATEFUL FOR
(I WILL TRY TO DO THIS EVERY DAY)

....
....
....
....

FUNNY THINGS YOU DID/SAID
(THANKS FOR MAKING ME LAUGH)

....
....
....
....
....
....
....
....
....
....
....
....
....
....

WHAT I WANT YOU TO KNOW
(YEARS FROM NOW)

....
....
....
....
....
....
....
....
....
....
....
....
....

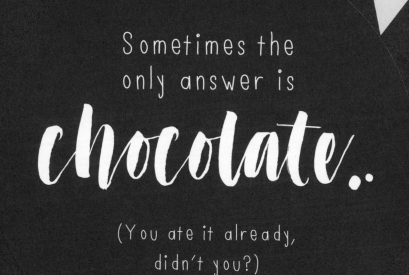

Sometimes the
only answer is

chocolate..

(You ate it already,
didn't you?)

ON THIS DAY

DATE: _____

Keep track of your cycle. It can really help to know WHY you're feeling the way you are.

MY NOTES
(WHAT I LOVED, FELT, WISHED, NEEDED, STRUGGLED WITH, OVERCAME)

....

....

....

....

....

....

....

....

TO DO LIST

❑ ....

❑ ....

❑ ....

❑ ....

❑ ....

YOU ARE YOUR THOUGHTS (SO MAKE THEM GOOD ONES)

LIFE DOESN'T HAVE TO BE HARD

How we think as adults is significantly different to how we thought when we were small. You only have to look at your child to realise just *how* different. Part of the frustrating reason why we can't get our kids to do the simplest of things *quickly,* like putting on their shoes, is because, in that moment, they're focused on something else; gratifying themselves with something they want to do *right* that minute. Something that makes them feel good and happy. Which, clearly, putting on shoes doesn't. They don't question that there might be any other way than this. When kids act up it's often because they are being prevented from doing the thing they *really* want to do – even if it is a) dangerous; b) massively inconvenient – and that makes them *really* cross. As grown-ups, we know we can't behave like this (at least not in public...). We can't throw our toys out of the pram to get what we want. But it goes deeper than this. Somewhere along the line, as we emerged from childhood, we began to hear from others that life is hard. That we must struggle to achieve whatever it is that we want. That *nothing* worth having comes easy. This message transports our thoughts and our efforts to a place of fear and self-doubt. Because, if it's *so* hard, what makes *us* so brilliant that we can rise to the challenge and succeed? Our minds become negative, anxious and scared, and they have the power to maroon us in a place we don't actually want to be, but where we stay because we are so afraid of failing.

THE POWER OF YOUR MIND

Every thought that passes through our mind manifests a response and a feeling, which influences everything we do and how we approach our lives. Living your life with frequent feelings of lack, anxiety and fear is joyless and frustrating, not to mention obstructive. It's the state of mind that stops us from being able to see the abundance in our lives, even though we *know* it is there. Yet, we never question the presence of negative thoughts. We've been conditioned to expect them and it feels much safer to trust in them than positive thoughts, which might amount to nothing and disappoint us. It's the same with those days, which we label as 'bad' and simply accept as our fate, in which one thing goes wrong after another. We perhaps don't see that it's only *us* who call them bad and who expect nothing less than one bad thing leading to another. But if one bad thing can lead to another, then surely one good thing can lead to another good thing, too? What if instead we choose to reframe the day, even after we've spilt the milk, missed the bus or shouted at everyone in the house? What about that nice conversation we had, which only came about because we missed that bus. Or the gift of the realisation that we'd prefer not to shout at our kids because it doesn't feel that good (even though, of course, we will again). It's what CBT calls 'challenging unhelpful thoughts'. And it totally works. With these kind of everyday annoyances, we *can* choose to see and feel them differently. Even when we're not feeling great, we can flip our mood and start to override those low moments and thoughts and attract the happy ones. We have that power. It just takes practice.

PURSUE THE FEELING NOT THE GOAL

So often in life, our mood is focused on and determined by an end goal. Often it's a significant milestone: marriage; a promotion and pay rise; having a baby; buying a bigger house with a garden and swing set. And so it goes on. This pursuit for what we perceive to be happiness never really ends when our focus is so driven and it's likely that we'll never be satisfied with whatever we achieve. What we often don't realise is that what we are going after isn't that specific 'success', but rather the feeling it brings: contentment, accomplishment, recognition, to name a few. But actually, those feelings are *not* exclusive to any one activity or major milestone and there are a million other, smaller ways of feeling those emotions that we crave so deeply, every day. The strange sense of achievement and satisfaction you get when you finally get around to eBaying all those clothes your child has grown out of. The happiness you're suddenly overwhelmed with when your child becomes a bit more self-aware and says or does something considerate and unexpected. The feeling of success when you serve up a home-cooked dinner and every plate at the end is clean. The recognition that comes when a colleague or client thanks you for helping them out of a tricky spot. None of these events are massive in themselves, but they can still give you the same feeling you sought from those larger 'life events'. The more of these feelings we experience, the more we learn about what makes us tick and the easier it is to nurture and recognise them day by day.

WHEN WE CAN'T TURN OUR THOUGHTS AROUND

Even the most positive-minded person hits a stumbling block, every now and then. Some days, no matter how much we try, no matter how much we *know* how to turn our mood around, we simply can't tune into the good thoughts. Sometimes it feels right at that moment to have a rant and a moan, even though we know this is more likely to attract the negative thoughts than the happy ones. That's ok. You're a busy mum with lots of demands on you and you're allowed to feel however you feel. So accept it and set about making just the next 10 minutes more pleasurable. Tick a small task off the to-do list. Conjure up a thought or memory that makes you happy. Have a treat – something delicious that you can really savour. Get some fresh air. Make a phone call to a friend. Anything that, when you think of it, raises your heart and lifts your mood. It won't take long to get back on track.

This moment
right now
is all you have.
Give it your
full attention.

ON THIS DAY

DATE: _____

Are you chasing a goal or a feeling? How else could you get that feeling?

MY NOTES
(WHAT I LOVED, FELT, WISHED, NEEDED, STRUGGLED WITH, OVERCAME)

....

....

....

....

....

....

....

TO DO LIST

☐ ....

☐ ....

☐ ....

☐ ....

☐ ....

THINGS TO REMEMBER
(THAT I'LL PROBABLY STILL FORGET)

....
....
....
....
....

WAYS I FEEL HAPPY
(ALL THE THINGS THAT RAISE MY HEART)

....
....
....
....
....

FUNNY THINGS YOU DID/SAID
(THANKS FOR MAKING ME LAUGH)

....
....
....
....
....
....
....
....
....
....
....
....
....

WHAT I WANT YOU TO KNOW
(YEARS FROM NOW)

....
....
....
....
....
....
....
....
....
....
....
....
....

you are your thoughts.

(So make them good ones.)

ON THIS DAY

DATE: _____

It's ok if you lose your way.
It's ok if it takes time to get back on track.

MY NOTES
(WHAT I LOVED, FELT, WISHED, NEEDFD, STRUGGLED WITH, OVERCAME)

....

....

....

....

....

....

....

....

....

....

....

TO DO LIST

❑ ....

❑ ....

❑ ....

❑ ....

❑ ....

50 REASONS WHY BEING A MUM ROCKS

For those days when you need a little reminder about why being a mum is so great, here it is. The definitive list of positive, optimistic, clutching-at-straws reasons why being a mum ROCKS.

1. There is always someone who loves you, unconditionally.
2. You care about 'all the other stuff' less then you did before.
3. You can do extraordinary things – and not just with frozen peas, pasta and cheese.
4. Fewer hangovers. Because there's less opportunity to go out.
5. Netflix.
6. You always have a reason for being late.
7. Or not turning up at all.
8. You get to play with cool stuff like Lego and Sylvanian Families.
9. And start sentences with, 'Can you please just put some pants on so...'
10. You have an excuse to listen to Justin Bieber and to watch all the new kids' films (even though you didn't need one).
11. Bedtime stories (with extra cuddles).
12. ALL the coffee.
13. ALL the gin.
14. ALL the biscuits.
15. ALL the cake.
16. You realise that nothing else really matters. As long as your child is happy and safe.
17. You become a world-class negotiator.
18. And multi-tasker.
19. You can go to cool places and do fun activities that you're way too old for.
20. You can lead a simpler life (if you let yourself).
21. You learn so much about yourself that you never knew before.
22. Mainly that you can do far more than you thought possible on much less (sleep).
23. This strength and resilience makes you as tough as a marine.
24. Whilst your child teaches you how to be more compassionate and empathetic.
25. Pyjamas are always an acceptable daytime outfit.
26. You cope. No matter what dramas life throws at you.

27. You're selfless every time you put your child first.
28. You're raising the astronauts, nurses and pioneers of tomorrow.
29. And shaping what the future looks like.
30. You might never have discovered dry shampoo.
31. You forget your troubles as soon as a small person nestles their head on your shoulder.
32. You get to live with Peppa Pig. A belly dancer. And a pirate. (Whilst dressing up yourself.)
33. You go to kids' theatre and enjoy it way more than your child.
34. You spend a lot more time outside, getting muddy or drinking up the sunshine. And it feels lovely.
35. Eventually you stop caring what other people think.
36. You give up trying to do things perfectly and realise that no one died.
37. You'll probably get a hamster.
38. The hamster will die.
39. You'll never have to get another one (the novelty wore off after three weeks).
40. More cake.
41. You make new friends and go through motherhood together.
42. They will get what you're saying before you've even said it.
43. You can explain your way out of ANYTHING.
44. You get to churn out the clichés that your own parents churned out.
45. You can post endless pictures of your child on Facebook and bore the pants off everyone.
46. Other people think you're amazing. (Because you are.)
47. You will never take sleep for granted, ever again.
48. Daytime naps – for you. Zzzzzzzzz.
49. You marvel at the person you've made. Every. Single. Day.
50. They're by far your biggest achievement. (Nothing else will ever come close.)

ON THIS DAY

DATE: _____

Do stuff that reminds you what happiness actually feels like.

MY NOTES
(WHAT I LOVED, FELT, WISHED, NEEDED, STRUGGLED WITH, OVERCAME)

....

....

....

....

....

....

....

TO DO LIST

☐ ....

☐ ....

☐ ....

☐ ....

☐ ....

THINGS TO REMEMBER
(THAT I'LL PROBABLY STILL FORGET)

....
....
....
....
....

WAYS I ROCK MOTHERHOOD
(BECAUSE I TOTALLY DO)

....
....
....
....
....

FUNNY THINGS YOU DID/SAID
(THANKS FOR MAKING ME LAUGH)

....
....
....
....
....
....
....
....
....
....
....
....
....

WHAT I WANT YOU TO KNOW
(YEARS FROM NOW)

....
....
....
....
....
....
....
....
....
....
....
....
....

The life of a *mother*
is one that's always
etched in *love.*

(And you're
doing it so well.)

ON THIS DAY

DATE: _____

You're raising a human being. What else comes close to that? Keep going.

MY NOTES
(WHAT I LOVED, FELT, WISHED, NEEDED, STRUGGLED WITH, OVERCAME)

....
....
....
....
....
....
....
....

TO DO LIST

☐ ....

☐ ....

☐ ....

☐ ....

☐ ....

BE A KICK A*** PARENTING TEAM

Motherhood. Fatherhood. Parenthood. Sometimes being parents together isn't easy or straightforward. There's way less time for you both, as a couple, and there's way more time for poor communication and misinterpretation. In tricky and tired moments (days, weeks or even months) when you feel out of sync with one another or can't feel the connection, it can be really difficult to be the formidable parenting team you actually are (and *you are*, by the way). Here are a few things that can be useful to remember when you're up against it (and one another). If you are a single parent, don't worry, there's a whole chapter coming up for you.

BE KIND TO ONE ANOTHER

This tops the list every time. It's simple. It's important. It can make up for a multitude of 'sins'. To be honest, it doesn't *really* matter if you or your other half occasionally forget to take out the bin, empty the dishwasher or do whatever chore it is you've agreed is yours. In hectic, tough times, things will get missed. You'll both feel stretched, and it's always nice to hear a kind word. To compliment one another. To feel your arms around one another. The odd bag of giant chocolate buttons totally doesn't hurt either.

TAKE OUT THE BIN

Ok, so I lied a bit above. It's always the little things, right? So try *not* to forget your chores.

HAVE SEX

Sex connects. It's what got you into this mess in the first place, remember? Also, some couples notice a direct correlation between the amount of times the bin gets put out and the amount of times *they* put out. Just saying. (More on this in the next chapter, in case you're a bit rusty).

DON'T COMPETE

It's the oldest parenting trap in the book and the most played out. Feeling the need to point out who's the most tired/frazzled/in demand. Don't. Go. There. You both are. So there are no winners here.

It's just a really crap game that makes you feel lousy. Get out the Scrabble instead, if you really need to do something competitive. Defuse everything with laughter – though it's tricky, this one, especially when you're finding it hard to find anything funny. But laughing is up there with sex. It makes you feel connected. Don't take it all too seriously. Parenthood won't always feel this hard or intense.

BE ON EACH OTHER'S SIDE

No one else is ever going to get your child like you both do. There is no one else who will love your child as much as you both do. So bond over how much you love them. Bond over how much you wish they'd just go to flipping sleep. Bond over how irritating it is that they've just had a meltdown in the middle of the supermarket and you had to abandon the trolley. But be on each other's side. Never blame one another. You're nurturing this person together. There *is* no one else to blame.

USE BANTER CAREFULLY

If you're a couple who liked to banter BC (before children), this can seriously backfire in early parenthood. Sometimes, the banter doesn't feel like a 'joke'. It feels more like a dig.

GO OUT TOGETHER

Going out together is important. Don't be that couple who wake up one day, realise that their kids are teenagers, and have nothing to talk about because they invested so little time in each other. If you don't want to go out/don't have a babysitter, have dinner at home together. Bottle of wine, conversation and no TV or phones. Or take the same day off work (if you work and that's possible). Oh and don't wait for the perfect time, or you'll be waiting forever. You deserve to put each other first every once in a while. Your partner might need this more than you – to have you all to themselves, for a change, and to feel what they still mean to you. No one said it has to be ALL about kids now, just because you're parents.

REMEMBER WHY YOU LIKED ONE ANOTHER

Focusing on that time before kids – and reliving those memories together – is a really good way of seeing yourselves through the challenging times. Go one better, remember the little gestures you did for one another and reinstate them when you can.

LOVE THE HELL OUT OF EACH OTHER

No explanation needed. Most couples, if not all, struggle at some point in their relationship, post-kids. But they usually get past it because they love each other. That, over and above everything else, makes ALL the difference.

things I love about my partner

....

....

....

....

....

Make time for
one another.
Your *love*
came first.

(Never take it for granted.)

ON THIS DAY

DATE: _____

Bond over your child. You're nurturing them together. How awesome is that?

MY NOTES
(WHAT I LOVED, FELT, WISHED, NEEDED, STRUGGLED WITH, OVERCAME)

....

....

....

....

....

....

....

....

....

....

TO DO LIST

❑ ....

❑ ....

❑ ....

❑ ....

❑ ....

THINGS TO REMEMBER
(THAT I'LL PROBABLY STILL FORGET)

....

....

....

....

....

MY 'COUPLES' WISH LIST
(HOW WE CAN SUPPORT ONE ANOTHER)

....

....

....

....

....

FUNNY THINGS YOU DID/SAID
(THANKS FOR MAKING ME LAUGH)

....

....

....

....

....

....

....

....

....

....

....

....

....

WHAT I WANT YOU TO KNOW
(YEARS FROM NOW)

....

....

....

....

....

....

....

....

....

....

....

....

....

Be on each
other's side.
ALWAYS.

(There's no one else's
side worth being on.)

ON THIS DAY

DATE: _____

Have fun
together.
LAUGH.

MY NOTES
(WHAT I LOVED, FELT, WISHED, NEEDED, STRUGGLED WITH, OVERCAME)

....

....

....

....

....

....

....

....

....

....

....

TO DO LIST

☐ ....

☐ ....

☐ ....

☐ ....

☐ ....

SEX AFTER KIDS ('ARE YOU HAVING A LAUGH?')

When I started thinking about this page, I had such a blank that I started writing about granola bars instead. Then a few fellow mums cheered me on: 'Sex? What's that? That's going to be a REALLY short section.'

DO YOU ACTUALLY NEED TO DO IT?

The short answer to this is 'YES'. The long answer is 'YES, you DO need to do it.' If you want to retain the intimacy of being a couple beyond being parents together, sex is important, and not just to men: women enjoy it too! That said, it's fair to say that post-kids, especially in the early years, even the randiest of couples find their sex life takes a hit, regardless of whether they still fancy the not-so-small pants off one another. It's a combination of lack of sleep, opportunity or the fact you've not slept in the same bed for 732 days.

FINDING THE OPPORTUNITY

Sometimes you've got to take out the romance and spontaneity and 'schedule' a rendezvous. Make it a verbal agreement – 'Shall we have sex tonight?'– rather than sending your partner a calendar invite. If you wait for the right time or to be in the mood, you may be waiting forever.

GETTING IN THE MOOD

Sex after a dry patch can be a bit, erm, awkward. Your conversation might be restricted to mundane topics like running out of nappies. So, TAKE IT SLOW. Don't go *all* out on the first few occasions and don a pair of crotchless knickers if you wouldn't have done this pre-kids. It doesn't have to be THAT considered. Setting the scene for LURVE these days means less sexy undies, candles and moody music and more wearing the not-so-grey-white pants and removing stray babies/toddlers/Kindles/digestives and anything else that has found its way into your bed.

'PLEASE DON'T TOUCH ME'

When you've been touched ALL day by a child and had ZERO personal space, the idea of getting intimate with your partner might horrify you. If this is the case, put some distance between yourself and the day. Ask them to do bedtime whilst you freshen up. A spritz of perfume and coat of lipstick can be a real mood-lifter, to remind you that you're also YOU (as well as someone's mum).

THE MOST FLATTERING SEX POSITIONS

Getting naked after babies can be scary. Getting naked AND sexual can be terrifying. You might be at peace with your post-baby body and not give a hoot who sees it – good for you! – or you might feel really self-conscious because things look and feel different. Do whatever makes you feel comfortable. Keep your bra on. Turn the lights down (or off). Have a glass of wine to relax you. Explain to your partner if you're feeling nervous; that usually breaks the ice. Whatever you do, don't try to recreate that bikini pose you saw that *really* sexy woman do on Instagram. She's not real.

WHEN ONE WANTS IT BUT THE OTHER DOESN'T

We're all frightened of being rejected. It's one of the reasons why couples give up on initiating sex, apparently – because they're fed up of being turned down. If there's discontent in how much sex you are (or aren't) having, talk. So often, a lack of desire originates from how unconnected one (or both) of you feels to the other. It's really normal in parenthood, when so much else is going on. Don't panic. It doesn't mean the attraction's gone, it just means you need to revive it. Talking and being tactile, on a daily basis, is the first step.

TAKING THE FUN OUT OF IT

If you're trying to conceive, sex can become a perfunctory activity, for both of you. That's ok. It's understandable. Just remember, it won't *always* be like this. Try to make it fun, whenever you can.

JUST DO IT

If ALL else fails, get on with it and take one for the team, so to speak. Because sex experts claim that the more sex you have, the more you want. This basically means that you have to do it to actually (hopefully) remember that you quite like it.

ON THIS DAY

DATE: _____

Sex connects.
So does
conversation.
Engage in both.

MY NOTES
(WHAT I LOVED, FELT, WISHED, NEEDED, STRUGGLED WITH, OVERCAME)

....

....

....

....

....

....

....

....

....

....

....

TO DO LIST

❑ ....

❑ ....

❑ ....

❑ ....

❑ ....

THINGS TO REMEMBER
(THAT I'LL PROBABLY STILL FORGET)

....
....
....
....
....

THINGS THAT TURN ME ON
(AND REASONS WHY I FIRST FANCIED YOU)

....
....
....
....
....

FUNNY THINGS YOU DID/SAID
(THANKS FOR MAKING ME LAUGH)

....
....
....
....
....
....
....
....
....
....
....
....

WHAT I WANT YOU TO KNOW
(YEARS FROM NOW)

....
....
....
....
....
....
....
....
....
....
....
....

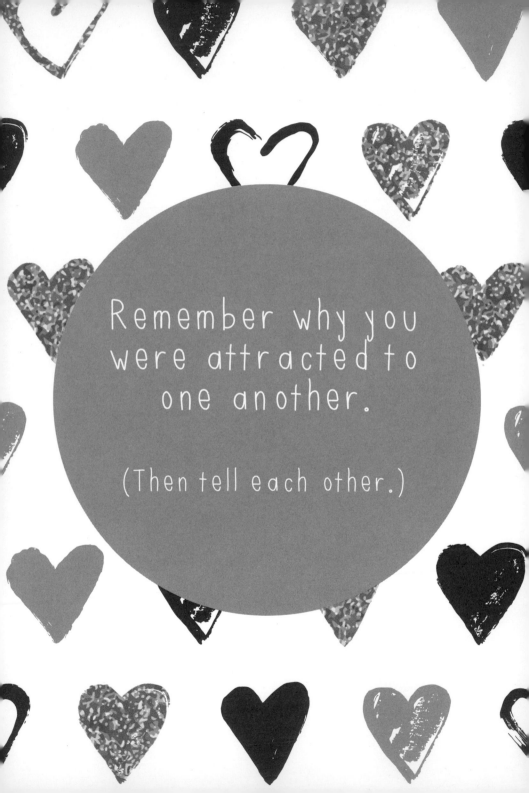

Remember why you were attracted to one another.

(Then tell each other.)

ON THIS DAY

DATE: _____

Do or wear
something that
makes you feel
SEXY.

MY NOTES
(WHAT I LOVED, FELT, WISHED, NEEDFD, STRUGGLED WITH, OVERCAME)

....

....

....

....

....

....

....

....

....

....

....

TO DO LIST

☐ ....

☐ ....

☐ ....

☐ ....

☐ ....

FLYING SOLO

YOU'RE AMAZING BECAUSE...

Parenting on your own, whether it's the result of separation or divorce, being widowed or because your partner works away or works long hours, is a HUGE achievement. Solo parents are HEROES. If you've separated from the other parent of your child(ren), this is never an easy, straightforward decision. Maybe it wasn't your decision at all. Having to be in contact with someone after the love has diminished – to continue raising your child(ren) together – can be painful and make the healing process longer. But you will heal – once you find a way to forgive and be around each other. Don't rush the process, but try to move beyond the past. Make a new vow between you: to always put your child(ren) at the centre of everything you do together. *You're amazing* because you'll do this, and it will make a huge difference to you all. If you've lost someone you love, I just want to say that I'm beyond sorry. *You're amazing* because you deal with your devastating grief but simultaneously find the strength, every day, to raise your child(ren) with grace, dignity and determination – likely without much of a break, ever. If you're solo parenting as a result of your other half's work location or because they work long days or on shift patterns, it's likely neither of you is finding this easy. The constant transition from solo parent to parenting couple and back to solo parent again is tough. *You're amazing* because you're both doing what you need to do for your family, even when that throws a curveball at the very thing you're trying to protect.

THE EMPOWERING SIDE OF SOLO PARENTING

The juggling involved when you're a solo parent can be really challenging – being both parents so much of the time. You might miss the shared responsibility of raising your kids, especially at bedtime, when bathing them and putting them to bed feels like climbing a mountain. Or in the middle of the night, when there is no one but you to deal with a wet bed, a nightmare, illness or a restless sleeper. Or at mealtimes when there's only you to get up 1,325 times to a) rescue a fork; b) take someone to the toilet; c) get someone a drink; d) rescue a spoon (slippery buggers, these cutlery items); e) catch that drink heading into a lap. You'll sometimes struggle with the sheer relentlessness of it all; with the juggling; with the guilt that occasionally seeps in, no matter how much you push it away. When tiredness hits and it causes you to be short-tempered with your child(ren), because there's nothing left in the fuel tank, remember that you are holding this s*** together. YOU. Just one person. And that makes you pretty amazing. That's the empowerment of solo parenting, right there. Showing you that you can totally do this shizzle (even when you think you can't). Please remember this when you're overtired, overwhelmed or hormonal and being touched/asked a question/touched again/whined at/ asked if you know where something is/hung off, etc. etc. etc. – and it all makes you want to lie down/sob/lie down some more/leave on a jet plane. Just look at all the things you are holding down! Be proud.

DON'T GIVE IN TO THE GUILT

The guilt of being a solo parent can eat you up, if you let it, regardless of whether it was your 'choice' or not. When your child is sad, struggling or something comes crashing down in their world, it is so easy to lose perspective and conclude that this can only be attributed to your situation. To blame yourself because you are supposed to make everything right in their world and you haven't. Stop – because kids in families with both parents have problems too. Kids are resilient. Also, it's never on us to fix *everything* in our kids' worlds. It's our role to support and guide them so they can see the way forward for themselves. You're already doing this every day, giving your kids an invaluable gift and defusing the outdated myth of what constitutes a 'normal' family unit. They will know that anything is possible, because of you. So keep believing in yourself, and in your path as a parent, which has led you here. Remember: there's nowhere else you can be but *right now*. Trust in the good times that are coming your way. Love your kids. And remember that guilt you often feel *always* comes from that love. Share a few words with someone else in your situation whenever you get the chance. It will ALWAYS make you feel better because no one else 'gets' it quite like another solo parent. And remember to be super kind to yourself. You are a really lovely and super special human being with SO much strength.

PRACTICAL TIPS FOR SOLO PARENTS

As a solo (separated) parent, I've learned that I need to take care of myself. That I can't be reckless with my well-being. So when I get some free time, I use it for me. NO GUILT – I've earned it and I need to recharge. I run. I read. I have a rebellious beer in the bath whilst listening to Madonna at full volume. I catch up on sleep. When the kids are with me I try to keep on top of things, but I also accept that there are days where I am overwhelmed and it's impossible. On these occasions, it's bagels and fruit for dinner on the sofa and I ground myself by snuggling in between the kids and reminding myself how lucky I am to have this much love (and chaos) in my life. Finally, I ALWAYS make our own rules. Because I refuse to maroon myself in a place where solo parenting is perceived as a tragedy. It isn't! My kids are loved by so many and our 'family' is a big, happy, eclectic mix of relatives and friends.

BEING THERE FOR SOLO PARENTS

If you're a friend of a solo parent, know that there are things you can do to support them. Simple tasks can be challenging when there's only one of you, so small gestures can make a huge difference. Offer to share the nursery run. Do an errand. Drop in with a coffee. Sit with their kid(s) so they can go for a run, pick up some milk or go out for the evening. Raising children by yourself can be really lonely, especially at the weekends when it's often all or nothing. Similarly, illness, when it strikes, can be isolating, especially when a child is ill with something contagious, such as chicken pox, and both parent and child are subjected to a week of quarantine. Or when the parent is unwell themselves and unable to get out. Checking in and letting them know you're there for them will help them face another day with a smile. And they will know that they're never alone.

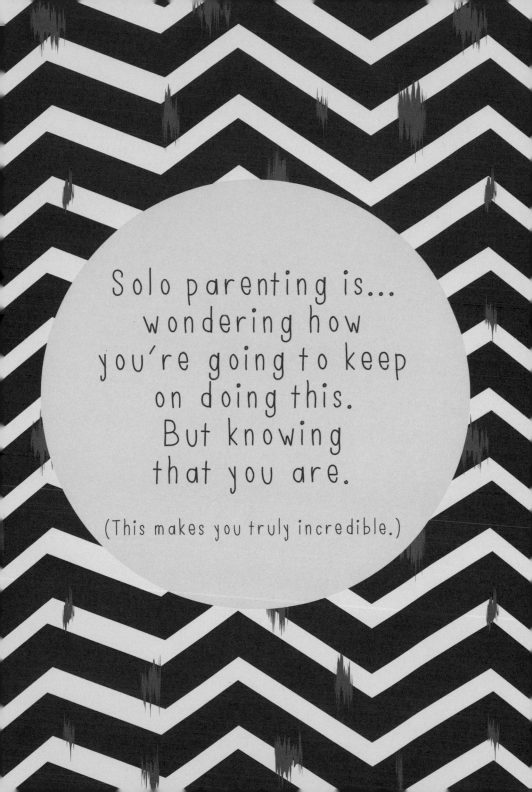

Solo parenting is...
wondering how
you're going to keep
on doing this.
But knowing
that you are.

(This makes you truly incredible.)

ON THIS DAY

DATE: _____

You're allowed to have feelings. It's ok if your child knows you get sad too.

MY NOTES
(WHAT I LOVED, FELT, WISHED, NEEDED, STRUGGLED WITH, OVERCAME)

....

....

....

....

....

....

....

TO DO LIST

☐ ....

☐ ....

☐ ....

☐ ....

☐ ....

THINGS TO REMEMBER
(THAT I'LL PROBABLY STILL FORGET)

....
....
....
....
....

'I AM AMAZING' CHECKLIST
(SO I CAN REMIND MYSELF OF ALL I HOLD DOWN)

....
....
....
....
....

FUNNY THINGS YOU DID/SAID
(THANKS FOR MAKING ME LAUGH)

....
....
....
....
....
....
....
....
....
....
....
....

WHAT I WANT YOU TO KNOW
(YEARS FROM NOW)

....
....
....
....
....
....
....
....
....
....
....
....

Try not to over-think
your situation.
Always *believe* you're
doing the best
you can.

(Because you are.)

ON THIS DAY

DATE: _____

Never forget how strong you are. Your strength is undeniable.

MY NOTES
(WHAT I LOVED, FELT, WISHED, NEEDED, STRUGGLED WITH, OVERCAME)

....

....

....

....

....

....

....

TO DO LIST

.... ❏ ....

.... ❏ ....

.... ❏ ....

.... ❏ ....

.... ❏ ....

HOW TO DO THE 'HOLIDAY DAYS' AS A FAMILY (CHRISTMAS, EASTER AND HALLOWEEN)

Ahhh. The wonderfulness of those oh so special holiday days. Especially when you mix up entertaining with nurturing small humans. Here's a few pointers, in case somewhere along the way you lose the will to live and need reminding what it's all about.

ROCK AN IMPERFECT FAMILY CHRISTMAS

Christmas. That most wonderful time of the year. Unless, of course, you heap on the pressure, stress yourself out with all the Christmas activities you simply MUST do and then cry because you've burned the turkey. A family Christmas will always be perfectly imperfect. Someone will have a meltdown. Someone else will cry. Something (many things) will go wrong. If you're hosting at a really high-pressured time, like Christmas Day, thinking of it as nothing more than a posh roast can help (because that's all it is). Also, remember that it really doesn't matter if the turkey is burned, or so dry that it falls off the bone in less of a tender way and more of a pencil shavings kind of way. Or that the Brussels sprouts are so undercooked they ping across the room when you try to put a fork in them. And you honestly don't need ten different kinds of sauces. Make it work for you, and everyone will be happier all round.

HOW TO DO A KICK-ASS EASTER EGG HUNT

Who doesn't enjoy an Easter egg hunt? Probably in the rain. First, remember to buy some little eggs. It's surprising how many people don't think to do this. Or totally forget that the 'odd one' they ate, while watching a box set, has actually amounted to 341. Oops. Next, get some nice Easter-themed baskets. Then forget where you put them, panic and use an old plastic bag with a hole in the bottom. Don't waste your time putting up direction signs. This is not an orienteering exercise. And your kids will lose any ability to focus when they hear the word 'chocolate'. Running around like headless chickens is the only technique they'll be using. Don't try to be clever and hide different-sized eggs, unless you want to spend the rest of the day listening to, 'It's not fair! Why are her eggs bigger than mine?' Don't bother putting your Easter Egg Hunt video on Facebook. It's crap. And no one needs to see your version of close-up soggy, blurred grass whilst you run around with an iPad. We've got our own. Let your kids eat all the eggs in one go, because why would you want to listen to 'Can we just have ONE more?' for the next month as you supervise their daily intake. Let them eat the lot and, who knows, if it makes them sick, maybe they'll go off chocolate forever. And then next year, you'll be spared running around like a loon whilst your childless neighbours look on in envy (pity).

HACK TOGETHER A HALLOWEEN PARTY

In recent years, Halloween has become really huge. My kids now demand a Halloween party after I got all excited and decided to throw one *once*. I remain in denial about this *every* year, then on the 31 October the guilt gets to me, I panic, invite anyone I can think of and put a party together in 3 hours. This basically involves hanging up last year's decorations (which are now, in fact, 10 years old), putting out a truckload of sweets and some skull-shaped crisps. If you succumb to pumpkins, get some really small ones, cut off the tops, hollow them out, rinse and fill them with cheesy pasta – with pumpkin pie on the side. The kids probably won't appreciate your efforts, but you'll get a rare flicker of what it's like to be a Pinterest Parent – and realise that it is totally (not) worth it. Top the afternoon off with some trick or treating, during which your children basically hassle your neighbours to give them even *more* sweets, and you'll pretty much have given your child the best day ever. And that is totally worth it.

ALWAYS KEEP IT SIMPLE

Whatever the occasion, if you're hosting actual people for an actual meal, this can feel really stressful when you're also raising small people (who will almost certainly want to hang onto your legs as you try to move around the kitchen to prepare). The guests will probably expect to eat something on a table not piled high with washing and stray (clean) pants. Arggghhh! The idea alone can feel overwhelming, especially if you've been out of the entertaining arena since having kids. The key here is to KEEP IT SIMPLE. Serve a meal that one of you can cook the night before (when meddlesome children are in bed), such as a lasagne (use the easy peasy recipe on page 215, if you like). Better still, cheat and buy something that looks fancy and transfer it to a ceramic dish. Or get your partner to remove your child(ren) from the house whilst you cook (transfer the lasagne and have a bath). Finally, serve loads of booze (something us parents are always good at doing) and no one will even care what they're eating anyway.

DON'T SUCCUMB TO PEER PRESSURE

Social media has a lot to answer for: perfect families ice-skating beautifully, and chuckling on the laps of Father Christmas (whilst yours recoiled and looked positively terrified), pictures of lovely, homemade, pastel-coloured Easter bonnets for organised Easter egg hunts with actual directions (which the children follow); kids in fields of orange with their wheelbarrows doing (the now obligatory) pumpkin picking. Your child will NOT be irreparably damaged if they don't do EVERY holiday activity going. Each time we've done *any* of these things, it's ended in a) injury; b) post traumatic stress disorder; and c) bankruptcy. The key here is to be sensible: do stuff you actually want to do and that is age-appropriate – and never let Facebook convince you otherwise.

OTHER PEOPLE'S EXPECTATIONS

Sometimes you can feel yourself dreading holiday days, as others heap their expectations upon you. You know what you *want* to do – focus on your little family – but other things can get in the way. You start to lose track of what's important or what's even reasonable and, before you know it, you're agreeing to something that makes you feel a little bit uneasy. It's never easy managing everyone else and their needs, especially at Christmas or Easter, with the expectations of extended family who we don't want to disappoint. As mothers, it becomes very natural to always try to please others, losing sight of our own desires and instincts in the process. I'm not sure anyone wins when we do this, so be the one who puts you all first, share your reasoning with your partner, be a united front and reach a decision that makes you *both* feel comfortable and content. Be fair and considerate and, if someone else doesn't like it, that is actually *their* problem, not yours.

FLYING SOLO ON HOLIDAY DAYS

If you're not with your kids at Easter, Christmas or any other typical 'family' occasion, because they're staying with the other parent, it's ok and perfectly normal to feel sad about this. Holiday days, when the world seems to be having the Best Time Ever (social media lies), can be really isolating. (In truth, they're probably bickering and trying to save the pencil-shaving turkey.) Have your own celebration with your child(ren) another time. Because it doesn't really matter *when* it happens, as long as it does. And how lucky is your little one to get two of these days? As for you? Try not to dwell on the fact that you don't have them with you. Make the best of it and host an amazing, stray-pant-free adult meal for family and friends or any other solo parents you know in the same boat.

SEE THINGS THROUGH YOUR CHILD'S EYES

The last time you got to see Christmas, Easter or Halloween through a child's eyes, you *were* one. Having your own children is an opportunity to feel the magic of these occasions again, to revisit all the old traditions of stockings, hidden chocolate and bobbing apples. When you find the pressure building, remember the joy of it all, and refocus your attention to what matters: your child (and you).

ON THIS DAY

DATE: _____

Forget about achieving perfection. It isn't necessary.

MY NOTES
(WHAT I LOVED, FELT, WISHED, NEEDED, STRUGGLED WITH, OVERCAME)

....

....

....

....

....

....

....

....

....

....

....

TO DO LIST

☐ ....

☐ ....

☐ ....

☐ ....

☐ ....

THINGS TO REMEMBER
(THAT I'LL PROBABLY STILL FORGET)

....
....
....
....
....

HOW TO ACE THE HOLIDAYS
(SHORTCUTS, TIME-SAVERS AND CHEATS)

....
....
....
....
....

FUNNY THINGS YOU DID/SAID
(THANKS FOR MAKING ME LAUGH)

....
....
....
....
....
....
....
....
....
....
....
....
....
....

WHAT I WANT YOU TO KNOW
(YEARS FROM NOW)

....
....
....
....
....
....
....
....
....
....
....
....
....

Nothing matters more than that **excitement** on your child's face. If what you're doing doesn't contribute to that, it doesn't need to be done.

ON THIS DAY

DATE:

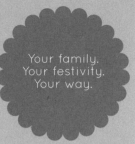

Your family.
Your festivity.
Your way.

MY NOTES
(WHAT I LOVED, FELT, WISHED, NEEDED, STRUGGLED WITH, OVERCAME)

....

....

....

....

....

....

....

....

TO DO LIST

❏ ....

....

❏ ....

....

❏ ....

....

❏ ....

....

❏ ....

EMERGING FROM THE EARLY YEARS (WHAT'S NEXT?)

NO MORE BABIES

The early years of motherhood are ALL-consuming, physically as well as mentally. As your child grows, becomes more independent and is able to do more for themselves, you will really start to see this, to appreciate just how *much* you've done and how much energy you've expended to get them to this point. If you're pregnant or planning more children imminently, you might not get the feeling that you're emerging, just yet. If, however, you're done having babies and it's almost time for your youngest/only child to start school, you might be feeling a little bereft/scared/'WHO ON EARTH AM I NOW?' Perfectly, perfectly normal. We all feel this. You – and they – are going to be just fine.

WHEN THE BABY BUBBLE BURSTS

The Baby Bubble is a bit like the Bermuda Triangle, but less exotic. And with more puke. Plus you never get to disappear completely, because there's always a small person tracking your *every* move. But you may feel that you've somehow been absent from the big wide world for a few years, and now your horizon is beginning to expand and you're ready to make a reappearance. It's different for all women, but for me it took a good couple of years to emerge from the bubble after my last baby. Not in some grand moment of glory, where I spread my beautiful painted wings and flew off into the sunset. More like a dusty old moth who'd eaten too many jumpers. If jumpers were, erm, McDonald's. Leaving the baby bubble is a bit of a shock. Because, as overwhelming as the baby bubble can be, especially in those early months, it's also a delightful little place that stops you having to think about what comes next. It stops you having to stand up and be counted. Wraps you in cotton wool, looks after you and hands you the TV remote, lots of caffeine and cake.

MOVING ON

Accepting that the procreation part of your life is over and getting back to any sort of normality after having your babies is weird and hard, especially if, up until this point, you've stayed at home to look after them. If you're not already back at work, what are you going to do next? After you've had a *really* long lie down, of course. Maybe you're working but have been putting off dealing with a job you no longer love because it suited the routine of those early years? Perhaps, as a working mum, you couldn't care less that the baby bubble has burst and are more concerned with the fact that soon you'll be juggling a job alongside way shorter school hours AND will somehow have to provide your child with an evening meal (schedules and tracking devices are your friend, I promise you). This new part of your life is all about being kind to yourself.

BUILDING A FORTUNE 500 COMPANY (AND FINDING CLEAN PANTS)

If you haven't been working, the void you're suddenly facing can be particularly unnerving. There are no more 'excuses' for not tackling all the to-dos you've been deferring, for not training for a marathon, for not reading all those books, for not organising all those photos. Now you've got all the time in the world to build that Fortune 500 company. And find some clean pants. EEK! Well, you know what? You *haven't* really got all the time in the world. Because the school day is short and by the time you've done the drop off, had a coffee and washed those pants, it will nearly be time to wend your way back to school again. BE KIND TO YOURSELF through this (and any) period of transition. Lots of us find change really difficult and it is totally fine to work your way through it gradually. It starts with small, forgiving steps. Allowing yourself some time to finally find a little headspace and use it for you, rather than someone else. Doing a bit of exercise because, actually, it makes you feel quite good, once you've silenced the voices in your head that have been telling you otherwise. Taking an art/baking/pottery/music/photography class, because you've always wanted to (and who knows where it might lead). Giving some thought to what you're putting into your body and taking the time to make that healthy brunch rather than that croissant you usually grab on the go. Opening yourself up to new opportunities and experiences that don't involve clapping your hands and nodding your head manically to 'If you're happy and you know it'. Feeling all the stuff, good and bad, until you reach that first flutter of excitement about your days not being all about babies or kids all of the time. Most importantly, it's now about YOU. Doing it (whatever 'it' is) in YOUR time. When YOU'RE ready. At YOUR own speed. There's no rush. And you're going to FLY.

Keep your
dreams
alive.

(Your time is always now.)

ON THIS DAY

DATE: _____

Always, always believe in yourself. You are marvellous.

MY NOTES
(WHAT I LOVED, FELT, WISHED, NEEDED, STRUGGLED WITH, OVERCAME)

....

....

....

....

....

....

....

....

....

....

....

TO DO LIST

☐ ....

☐ ....

☐ ....

☐ ....

☐ ....

ON THIS DAY

DATE: _____

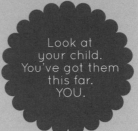

Look at your child. You've got them this far. YOU.

MY NOTES
(WHAT I LOVED, FELT, WISHED, NEEDED, STRUGGLED WITH, OVERCAME)

....

....

....

....

....

....

....

....

TO DO LIST

☐ ....

☐ ....

☐ ....

☐ ....

☐ ....

THINGS TO REMEMBER
(THAT I'LL PROBABLY STILL FORGET)

....

....

....

....

....

WHAT I MIGHT LIKE TO TRY NEXT
(THINGS THAT MAKE ME FEEL BUTTERFLIES)

....

....

....

....

....

FUNNY THINGS YOU DID/SAID
(THANKS FOR MAKING ME LAUGH)

....

....

....

....

....

....

....

....

....

....

....

....

....

WHAT I WANT YOU TO KNOW
(YEARS FROM NOW)

....

....

....

....

....

....

....

....

....

....

....

....

....

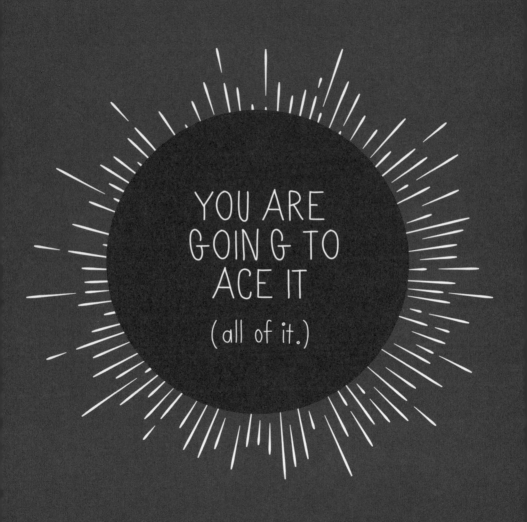

YOU ARE
GOING TO
ACE IT

(all of it.)

A POEM FOR YOU, AN AMAZING MUM

There's more to you than meets the eye
More than nappies and crumbs
You've got dreams and needs all of your own
Beyond being somebody's mum.

'You're lucky' to have them, you know, you know
But sometimes you just want to scream,
To dig out some heels and get out on the town
And start pursuing those dreams.

It's ok to admit how hard it can be
When the days stretch endlessly ahead
And the tantrums, tears and constant demands
Make you wonder why you got out of bed.

'You wouldn't change it,' blah blah blah
Except that sometimes you would.
You'd swap it all, just for a moment,
For the life you once knew, if you could.

It changes you, becoming a mum,
Nothing can be what it was
Those frivolous days are a thing of the past
Everything comes at a cost.

But the price that you pay is never too much
For those small people you hold in your heart
You love them to the moon and right back
And you could never bear being apart.

So today as you sweep the floor yet again
And wipe yet another nose
Remember now how amazing you are
And how quickly these days will go.

A CLOSING LETTER TO
A NOT-SO-NEW MUM

Dear Not-So-New Mum,

So, here we are. Maybe 2 or 3 years on from when you first started noting things down in this book. Older and wiser. Stronger and resilient. Kinder and more empathetic. Probably still a bit tired.

I have enjoyed writing this notebook more than I can tell you. To be able to share the little things that I've learned, that have made a BIG difference to my life as a mother, has been such a privilege. Thank you for reading it and letting me walk alongside you. I hope that it has helped you feel better, when you've needed to.

As this book is published, my youngest and final 'baby' starts school. This feels like no coincidence to me and it is the perfect conclusion to *my* early years. There are, of course, so many more to come, but nine years of looking after my three young in our nest has – as everyone said it would – gone by in a flash. I'm glad I occasionally took the time to *really* notice them, the ordinary moments and myself.

I know, of course, that when you're going through it, and some days are tough, that it doesn't feel like a flash - at all. It can feel long and exhausting and like it will *never* get easier. I hope this notebook will always show you *how far* you've travelled. Remind you of the things you overcame and the happy moments that are now beautiful memories. Because the passing of time certainly dissolves the difficult moments we went through and is most definitely the reason I now often find myself nostalgically watching a mum with her baby or a toddler in tow, and feeling so moved by her presence. Isn't she amazing? If there are no more babies in your future, I'm sure you do this too.

If your 'early years' aren't yet over and there's another baby following in the shaky steps of your first intrepid toddler, I know that you will find the years that follow to be easier in some ways and harder in others. Your first experience of being a mother is new and uncertain. We certainly benefit from experience and the ability not to sweat the small stuff. Of course, having a bigger tribe to nurture is tiring. Encourage each of your children to feel a *real* member of that tribe, to discover their place and to take some small responsibility and pride in being a part of it. Watching mine begin to do this has been so wonderful. It's what I believe we're meant to do in our role as mothers: guide, not control.

The journey of a mother is an epic one. There is nothing that we will *ever* do that will even come close to this. Of that, I am sure. To raise a small person (or people) is *such* a responsibility, but it is also *such* an honour. Helping to shape a mind, a personality and a future is something that deserves our awe and wonder every single day. And it's not necessary to martyr ourselves to do this incredible thing. Those little minds and personalities we're shaping are never ours to own. They are free and spirited and only require the security of our love to reach their potential. Because when our kids are loved, when they are believed in and encouraged, they can do anything they put their minds to.

> 66 The journey of a mother is an epic one. There is nothing that we will ever do that will even come close to this. 99

Finally. YOU. The amazing woman behind the mother; the woman who came *long* before the mother ever did. I hope that you see how happy you deserve to be, how fulfilled. And that you *also* believe that you can do anything you put *your* mind to.

Always remember: the journey is your own. And I wish you all the love and happiness in whatever comes next in yours.

Amy x

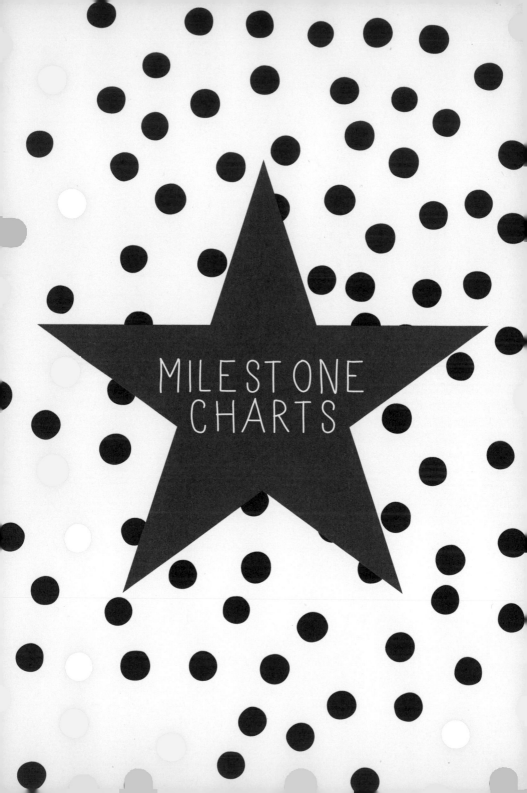

MILESTONE
CHARTS

I wish I could remember when my child...

Use these charts to keep a record of your child's milestones. And your own. (Because you will forget them.) Just pop the date and milestone in the box – there are almost enough for one a week.

Year One

Year Two

Year Three

Year Four

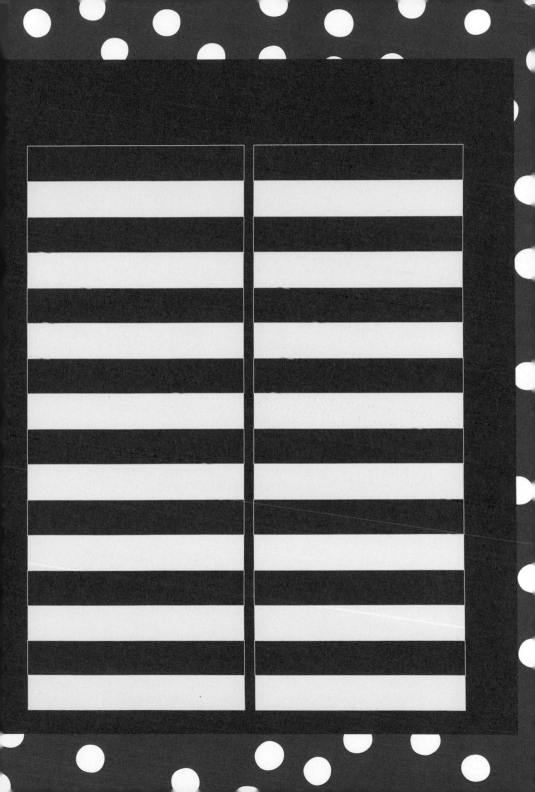

NOTES

NOTES

NOTES

NOTES

NOTES

NOTES

NOTES

NOTES

NOTES

ACKNOWLEDGEMENTS

There are a few people I would like to thank, whose friendships and spirits alone enable me to do this 'writing books' (and general life) lark. I'll try and keep it brief.

To Gina, I'm *so* glad you took on the design (again)! You give this Notebook series life and your passion makes it so easy and fun working with you. My dear friend, Luce. Thank you for everything; you will never be rid of me, so please stop trying. To Dace, you are one of the best things to come out of my separation. Thank you for always shining your light (and logic) in my path. To my amazing friend and mum of six, Sarah; you have inspired so much of this book and the life I now choose to live, as myself and a mother. To Victoria, thank you for the playgroup years and all the positive encouragement – I can't believe this part of my life is over! To Sarah, Anneli, Sam, Sujeeta, Charlotte, Ellie, Tom, Lynne and everyone at The Nursery on the Green (past and present), thank you so much for helping me raise three happy children (and almost doing a better job than me!). To my inimitable mum, dad and sister, you always let me be myself and find my own way, which I am discovering is all we ever need to do as parents and people. To all my single-parent friends navigating this tricky terrain, thanks for getting it. All of it. Keep going and, when you can't keep going, lean back until you can once more. To Trevor, for taking so much interest in all that I do, always being strong enough to shield me from the rain and reading this book as I wrote it. To my agent, Laura, and my publisher, Sarah, thank you for working with me to get another beautiful notebook out there.

Finally, to my three lovely children. Thank you for all the life lessons. Having a book published was always my dream and now here I am with two. Yet you show me, every day, that success doesn't lie in what we do (or don't) achieve. It's in much smaller and simpler acts than that. It's in all the glorious, ordinary moments that are right in front of us, if we just step back enough to notice them. And I count myself so lucky to share these with you. Never doubt that you're whole, that you matter or that you're worthy. As you are.

 x